P9-BYW-724

A WOMAN'S GUIDE TO VITAMINS, MINERALS, & ALTERNATIVE HEALING

SHERRY WILSON SULTENFUSS, M.S. &
THOMAS J. SULTENFUSS, M.D.

MJF BOOKS
NEW YORK

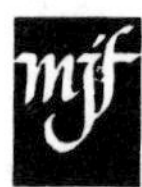

Published by MJF Books
Fine Communications
Two Lincoln Square
60 West 66th Street
New York, NY 10023

A Woman's Guide to Vitamins, Minerals, and Alternative Healing
ISBN 1-56731-407-4
LC Control Number 00-135235

This edition published by arrangement with Contemporary Books, an imprint of NTC/Contemporary Publishing Group, Inc.

Manufactured in the United States of America on acid-free paper

10 9 8 7 6 5 4 3 2 1

THIS BOOK IS dedicated to our mothers, Margaret and Agnes; our daughters, Katherine and Margo; all women taking responsibility for their health; and the thousands of researchers and practitioners who have dedicated their lives to the betterment of ours.

Contents

Preface vii
Acknowledgments ix
1 Introduction 1

I **The Hows and Whys of Vitamin and Mineral Supplements** 5

2 Vitamins and How to Buy Them 7

II **The Inside Story on Nutritional Supplements** 15

3 Vitamin A 17
4 The B Vitamins 23
- Thiamine (B_1) 24
- Riboflavin (B_2) 25
- Niacin (B_3) 26
- Pantothenic Acid (B_5) 28
- Pyridoxine (B_6) 29
- Folic Acid 30
- Cyanocobalamin (B_{12}) 32
- Biotin 34
- Para-Aminobenzoic Acid (PABA) 34
- Inositol 35
- Choline 36

5 Vitamin C 37
6 Vitamin D 43
7 Vitamin E 47
8 Vitamin K 55
9 CoQ_{10} 59
10 Boron 63
11 Calcium 65
12 Chromium 71
13 Copper 75
14 Iodine 77
15 Iron 79
16 Magnesium 83
17 Manganese 87
18 Molybdenum 89
19 Phosphorus 91

20 Potassium 93
21 Selenium 95
22 Zinc 99

III Topics of Prime Concern to Women **101**

23 Bones 103
24 Cancer 113
25 Estrogen and Hormone Replacement Therapies 123
26 Exercise 131
Optimizing Aerobic Exercise Intensity
Robert Greenwell, M.D. 137
27 Fish Oils 147
28 Food
Nan Jensen, R.D., L.D., and Phil Hanna 151
29 The Female Heart 171
30 Herbs 177
31 Menopause 185
32 Premenstrual Syndrome (PMS) 191
33 Skin and Aging 195
Laser Resurfacing for the Treatment of Facial
Wrinkles and Scars
Susan S. Roper, M.D. 212
34 Weight 217

IV Alternative Therapies **223**

35 Acupuncture, Herbs, and Traditional Chinese Medicine
Mary Felicia Bochichio, A.P., D.A., Dipl. Ac. 225
36 Chiropractic
Scott L. Drizin, D.C., M.P.S., F.A.A.B.T.,
and Ellen C. Drizin, M.S. 237
37 Osteopathic Medicine
Larry Horvath, D.O. 245
38 Allopathic Medicine: Traditional Western Medicine
Thomas Sultenfuss, M.D. 249

V Putting It All Together **253**

39 Recommendations 255

Notes 263
Index 311

Preface

Rewriting this book gave me a chance once again to become totally absorbed in medical and nutritional literature. In 1995, when we wrote the first book, there was a scarcity of information relating to the health needs of women over the age of 18. Few studies that included women existed, and little information was available that pertained to optimal ranges necessary for vitamins, minerals, and herbs. I am pleased to say that in 1998 so much more information is available. Many more researchers are focusing on individual vitamins, minerals, and herbs to ascertain the optimal levels necessary for good health and what each one is "good" for.

I also saw more of a meeting of the minds between traditional and nontraditional practitioners. Each appears to be a little more accepting of the other, and more information seems to be traded between them. We are not truly "integrated" in our health care yet, but we are making positive strides.

Sherry Wilson Sultenfuss

Acknowledgments

KAREN ROTH, M.L.S., medical librarian: Thank you so much for all your help and for being so nice and always cheerful.

We would also like to thank the following people for their invaluable help reviewing and editing sections of the book. It would have been lacking without each and every one of them.

Mary Tahan, book agent
Linda Nichols Beyrouti, R.P.T., physical therapy
Mary Felicia Bochichio, A.P., D.A., Dipl. Ac., Chinese medicine and acupuncture
Gene Brissie, editor of the first edition
Scott L. Drizin, D.C., M.P.S., F.A.A.B.T., chiropractic
Ellen C. Drizin, M.S.
Erika Lieberman, editor of the revised edition
Robert Greenwell, M.D., sportsmedicine and cardiac rehabilitation
Phil Hanna, creative input
Larry Horvath, D.O.
Nan C. Jensen, R.D., L.D., nutrition
Mitchell Lowenstein, M.D., rheumatology
Patrice A. Moreno, M.D., cardiology
Louis Paolillo, M.D., obstetrics and gynecology
Susan Roper, M.D., dermatology
Charles Yamokoski, D.O., oncology

I

Introduction

We rewrote this book, updating the scientific literature on vitamins, minerals, and herbs, to help the over-18-year-old, healthy, nonpregnant woman. We have also included the expertise of practitioners who have shared some of their medical knowledge. Hopefully this review will arm women with enough information to make intelligent decisions on nutritional choices, vitamin and mineral supplements, and medical options for "optional health."

Section I is an overview of vitamins and minerals and how to purchase them. Section II contains information on many of the most common vitamins, minerals, and herbs, and how they affect most women. Section III provides information on bones, cancer, estrogen and hormone replacement therapies, exercise, fish oil, food, heart, herbs, menopause, PMS, skin, laser resurfacing, and weight. Section IV explores Chinese acupuncture, chiropractic, osteopathic, and traditional medical doctors. Section V lists the most recent *recommended dietary, or daily allowances* (RDAs) of vitamins and minerals, their best chemical form(s) and toxicity levels, and summarizes the recommended ranges of the vitamins and minerals from the reviewed literature. Also included is a summary of nutritional recommendations from the research.

An estimated 70 percent of all Americans take some form of dietary supplement. It is approximately a $4 billion gross sales industry.[1] Yet some say that the efficacy of supplements still has not been proven effective and question their safety.[2] A large epidemiological study conducted in Finland of 5,100 women and men taking supplements showed positive health results in the people with the highest vitamin intake. The women with the highest intake of vitamins, whether through diet or supplementation, showed the highest reduction risk for cardiovascular disease.

We need to be aware of the magnitude of the health care industry today. It is one of the largest industries and will continue to grow as baby boomers age. Bad-mouthing traditional M.D.'s has become commonplace. However, just as in any field, there are the good, the bad, and the ugly. "Alternative" physicians can't cure all the ills of the world either. They all need to work together since each has an important part to play.

I am pleased to see the integration of mainstream and alternative medicine that has taken place in the past three years in research and practice. Traditional medicine is expanding its research into nutrition and prevention, and alternative health care providers are demanding more accountability from themselves. Our job is to wade through it all and find the best solutions for ourselves. My only real concern for the future is not for the method of cure or the medical professionals, because I believe we are on a positive track, but for our health care system. I am concerned that it may restrict our medical choices and future research. We need to be proactive not only for our own health concerns but for the good of everyone.

A recent study estimated the reduction in hospital costs through vitamin supplementation. It estimated that $20 billion could be saved by the use of supplementing with folic acid, zinc, and vitamin E. Folic acid and zinc would help women of child-bearing years to prevent birth defects and low birth weight babies. Supplementation with vitamin E, for those over 50, could help to reduce coronary artery disease. It was estimated that 70 percent of health care costs are preventable.[3]

As laypeople we must rely on our judgment based on common sense and research to choose the best nutritional diet, supplementation program, and medical care. We should be wary of fads and companies that make remarkable claims to fix our health problems. We must be careful not to overdose ourselves on any vitamins, minerals, or herbs, or be blindly led by health practitioners. It is imperative when taking a supplement to balance the components. They can interact with one another, and some combinations and dosages may be synergistically beneficial or harmful. Evidence shows that taking large doses of one vitamin or mineral can cause a deficiency in another. For example, large doses of zinc increases the loss of copper and iron. It is also imperative to let all health practitioners know all supplements, herbs, traditional medications, and therapies that you are taking. They are all chemicals that interact with one another.

Fortunately, many more research dollars are now being allocated to the study of vitamins, minerals, and herbs. In a few more years, the results of some large long-term studies will be completed and new insights will unfold. Hopefully this will settle many disputes. But until then, it is up to each of us to make smart choices.

This book is not a medical text. It is a review of some of the scientific literature. No prescriptions are given. The nutritional and medical suggestions in the book are collated from many researchers, physicians, and nutritionists. Many of the studies reviewed are controversial, and the conclusions may be disputed. The sources of information are mostly from medical and nutritional journals.

To contact the authors, please visit www.awomansguide.com or call 877-UR-GUIDE.

Part I

The Hows and Whys of Vitamin and Mineral Supplements

2

Vitamins and How to Buy Them

Are Supplements Necessary?

VITAMINS, ORGANIC COMPOUNDS found in plant and animal food sources, are necessary *in small amounts* for health and maintenance of body tissues. They must be present in the diet or in supplements since the human body cannot manufacture them. *Hormones* also are needed in small amounts for the same general purposes, but they are manufactured in the body. *Minerals* are naturally occurring, inorganic substances.

An argument has raged for years over the nature and definition of a vitamin. The key to the argument is the phrase *in small amounts*. Recommended vitamin dosages have been defined in the past as the dosages necessary to prevent specific deficiency diseases such as scurvy, pellagra, beriberi, and rickets. But are these the dosages needed for optimal health? At higher dosages, do vitamins have benefits other than the prevention of deficiency diseases? Recent research has some fascinating if incomplete answers to these questions, as we will see in later chapters.

Vitamins A, E, D, and K are *fat-soluble* vitamins and are stored in fatty tissues and in the liver. The other vitamins are *water soluble* and are stored in the body for a few hours to several days. Quite a bit of controversy exists about taking vitamin and mineral supplements. Some people think that we get all the necessary nutrients from a well-balanced diet; others feel that the American diet in general is nutritionally incomplete. One reason claimed is that the soil that supports both plant and animal life has become somewhat depleted of essential minerals, often due to long-term erosion of farmland. Another reason offered is that modern processing and milling of foods removes much of the vitamin and mineral content.

Whether a person chooses to take a daily vitamin and mineral supplement or not, it is important to eat a well-balanced, varied diet, drink plenty of fluids, limit calories for a specific body size, get plenty of rest (without stress), and exercise regularly. Writing about the above five requirements is all too easy, yet fitting them into a busy life is so difficult. A vitamin and mineral supplement ideally will act, just as intended, as an aid to our present and future health. Vitamins are not a cure-all, nor should they be used as a stimulant to give energy or as a substitute for a well-balanced diet.

The *recommended dietary, or daily allowances*, (RDAs) established by the Food and Nutrition Board of the National Research Council of the National Academy of Sciences are designed as guidelines to ensure that most of a healthy population is meeting its nutritional needs. Remember, however, that the RDAs are not designed for individuals but for populations. Other groups such as the World Health Organization, the Food and Agriculture Organization, and governmental agencies of many individual countries also have nutritional recommendations. These different groups do vary in their guideline estimations and recommendations.[1] However, much of the recent scientific literature suggests that in many cases the RDAs are not adequate for optimal health. The recommendations may simply ward off deficiencies rather than enhance health.

Do Women Need to Take Vitamin and Mineral Supplements?

Our bodies need approximately 40 different nutrients in order to maintain good health. Traditional medical wisdom once said that all the necessary vitamins and minerals can be obtained in a well-balanced diet. But researchers can provide evidence that women need vitamin and mineral supplementation if they are smoking, nursing, dieting, under stress, or pregnant, are heavy menstrual bleeders, vegetarians, or have gastrointestinal problems.[2] A large-scale nutritional study on both men and women found that both girls and women were at the highest risk of low intakes for the 11 minerals analyzed. Calcium, magnesium, iron, zinc, copper, and manganese were low, less than 80 percent of the listed RDAs.[3] In another two-year study, about 70 percent of the women studied consumed less than 70 percent of the RDAs for both zinc and folic acid. Another 30 percent of the women took in less than 70 percent of the RDAs for calcium and iron. And 40 percent of the women had inadequate intake of B_6 and magnesium.[4]

Many vitamin deficiencies may increase the risks for some diseases and speed up the aging process. These adverse effects may be partly due to free-radical reactions. A *free radical* is a highly reactive atom or molecule with an unpaired electron. The unpaired electron can cause damage to fats, structural proteins, enzymes, and informational macromolecules, such as DNA. This free-radical damage can be reduced by antioxidants such as beta-carotene, vitamin C, vitamin E, and selenium.

The free radical theory was first introduced in 1954 by Dr. Denham Harman. He proposed that cells have built-in protective enzymes that can either detoxify free radicals or correct the damage done by them. In the process of aging, the enzymes can no longer keep up with the damage being done, and breakdowns in the system occur. This process can be compared to leaving fatty food out on a table overnight. Oxygen reacts with the food and turns it rancid. This is similar to the damage done in the body by free radicals. The free radicals attack the body's cells internally and start deterioration. Antioxidants lessen this free-radical damage.

How to Buy a Vitamin and Mineral Supplement

So many vitamin and mineral supplements flood the market that buying one intelligently seems an overwhelming task. It is difficult enough to decide which supplements are needed without being confused by the various labeling formats. It is imperative to read the labels and to understand them.

Understanding Labels

An ingredient listed on the label may be listed plainly, or part of it may be in parentheses. The two listings mean very different things. For example, if the item is zinc picolinate, it can read as zinc picolinate 50 mg or zinc (picolinate) 50 mg. In the first example, 50 milligrams (mg) is the combined weight of the zinc and the picolinate. In the second example, 50 mg refers to the weight of the elemental zinc and does not include the weight of the other part in parentheses (picolinate). So if you want to take 50 mg of zinc, pick the second example.

The "Other Ingredients"

Bioavailability of a vitamin or mineral refers to how efficiently it is absorbed by the body. Minerals are usually compounded with other substances that affect bioavailability. This compounding process of binding other substances to the vitamins and minerals is called *chelation.*

Back to the example of zinc picolinate. The zinc is chelated with picolinate to make the zinc easier to absorb (more bioavailable). There are three basic types of chelation: inorganic mineral salts, organic mineral chelates, and full-range amino acid chelates. The inorganic mineral salts are usually oxides, phosphates, and carbonates. The organic mineral chelates usually employ fumarates, gluconates, citrates, and different amino acids. The full-range amino acid chelates are very complex. This new form supposedly presents minerals in their most bioavailable form.

However, opinions differ as to which process is superior. In some cases the organic mineral chelates and the full-range amino acid chelates appear more bioavailable. This greater absorption is due to a change in the electrical charge of the chelated minerals. The organic mineral and full-range amino acid chelates are also generally more expensive.[5] Despite doubts by some that the investment in chelated mineral supplements is worthwhile,[6] other authorities are enthusiastic about their benefits outweighing their cost.[7, 8]

There are many *antagonists*, or substances that inhibit the absorption of a vitamin or mineral. How these substances act depends on the vitamin, mineral, or combination taken and how it is taken. Regardless of this chelate debate, having a *balanced* vitamin and mineral supplement is important. Tissue damage and deficiencies can result from taking the inappropriate dosages or combinations.

Some vitamin and mineral supplements contain many other ingredients, including food coloring, preservatives, binders, and fillers. Many of these may cause other problems such as allergies or other physical reactions. We do not know how these other ingredients may react with the body when taken over a long period of time.[9] The problem of hidden ingredients will be eliminated by new Food and Drug Administration (FDA) regulations mandating the listing of both active and inactive ingredients.

Natural Versus Synthetic

An undying controversy continues over the supposed advantages of natural versus synthetically derived vitamins. Some authorities claim natural vitamins are superior, and others say that it really doesn't make any difference. Generally the natural ones are more expensive. We found little actual scientific research available on this topic, but this is probably due to the rather obvious argument that if two vitamin molecules are identical, their origins are irrelevant. An ascorbic acid (vitamin C) molecule has no ancestral memory to tell it whether it came from an orange or a test tube. Vitamin E (tocopherols) from natural sources has generally been regarded as being more potent than synthetic vitamin E, but this is because the synthetic form is sold as a mixture rather than pure d-alpha tocopherol.

Many of the natural vitamin preparations also include other ingredients, which, depending on the item, may also be beneficial. For example, rose hips include not only vitamin C but also flavonoids, fructose, malic acid, sucrose, tannins, zinc, vitamins A1, B3, D, and E.

Expiration Dates and Regulations

Check the expiration date! Vitamin and mineral supplements can lose their potency quickly. Many of them are sensitive to light, heat, oxygen, and moisture. According to current regulations, only 90 percent of the potency listed on the label has to be present at the time of shipping. Manufacturers are presently required by the government to do very little shelf-life testing, and some manufacturers exercise little laboratory quality control.

When and How to Take a Vitamin and Mineral Supplement

Although following the directions on the label is important, it appears better to take a vitamin and mineral supplement three times a day rather than all at once. The water-soluble vitamins have a greater chance to be absorbed and used if they are taken at intervals throughout the day rather than all at once. Time-release vitamins also appear to be of value. They slowly release the ingredients into the body throughout the day.

Weight Equivalents

Unit	Equivalency
Kilogram (kg)	1,000 g
Gram (g)	1,000 mg
Milligram (mg)	1,000 mcg
Microgram (mcg)	1,000 ng
Nanogram (ng)	1,000 picogram (pg)

Units of Measurement of Vitamins

Vitamin	Unit of Measurement	Definition
A	Retinol Equivalent	1 mcg of all-trans retinol 6 mcg of all-trans beta-carotene 12 mcg of other provitamin A carotenoids

D	International unit (IU)	Equivalent to the activity of 0.025 mcg of cholecalciferol
E	International unit (IU)	Equivalent to the activity of 1 mg of the acetate form of dl-alpha tocopherol.

Checklist for Buying a Vitamin/Mineral Supplement

1. Know what supplements you want and why you want to take them.
2. Check the ingredients and the presence of parentheses for ingredient amounts.
3. Look out for preservatives, coloring agents, fillers, and binders.
4. Check the expiration date.
5. Take the supplement as directed.
6. Do not take megadoses of vitamins without a doctor's supervision.

Part II

The Inside Story on Nutritional Supplements

3

Vitamin A

Primary Functions

Prevents night blindness and other eye disorders
Keeps skin moist and elastic, including the eyes and vagina
Maintains healthy hair, skin, gums
Reduces risk of breast cancer*
Helps alleviate *mastodynia*, sore breasts*
May reduce the risk of lung cancer*
Maintains cell structure and integrity[1]
Works as an antioxidant to prevent cell aging and possibly atherosclerosis[2]*
Helps prevent infection[3]
Derivatives of vitamin A treat acne, fine skin wrinkling, and the effects of sun damage

Night blindness was recognized as a disease centuries ago by the early Egyptians, but not until this century was the preventative agent found to be a fat-soluble compound present in egg yolks, butter, and fish oil.[4] Today vitamin A is the subject of many different and varied research projects, including its possible value in reducing a woman's risk of breast cancer.

*Higher levels of vitamin A as beta-carotene

Vitamin A is a fat soluble vitamin. The term *vitamin A* is used to include retinol and a group of chemically similar compounds referred to as *retinoids*. They are found in animal products and are toxic at high dosages. Vitamin A as *beta-carotene* is found mostly in fruits and vegetables and is not toxic at any known dose. Beta-carotene is a provitamin; it is only turned into retinol as the body requires. Beta-carotene is probably at least as important as retinol in maintaining health.

Some interesting links have been shown between beta-carotene plasma levels and the occurrence of cancer [5,6] and heart disease. It is known that beta-carotene is a powerful antioxidant that protects membranes from free-radical damage, while retinol strongly influences epithelial tissue (skin, membrane, lining of internal organs) growth.[7] In one study, beta-carotene, not retinol, was thought to be a protective agent against myocardial infarction (heart attack).[8] It also has been suggested that beta-carotene, and not retinol, may be a protective factor against breast cancer. A New York study, examining 439 postmenopausal breast cancer patients, found that the risk was highest in women who had low intakes of beta-carotene. Retinol was not considered a risk factor.[9] On the other side of the world, in Moscow, researchers came to similar conclusions. They found that people who consumed large amounts of animal products were at greater risk for breast cancer. Individuals who had high intakes of fruits and vegetables had a low risk for breast cancer.[10] In Singapore similar results were found, but only in premenopausal women. This case-controlled study of 200 patients with breast cancer indicated that the high risk factor for cancer was a high consumption of red meat. The low risk factor for cancer was a high consumption of dietary protein from soybean products, high intakes of polyunsaturated fats, and high intake of beta-carotene.[11]

Retinol normalizes the maturation of epithelial tissues and therefore is usually thought to have a protective effect against epithelial cancers. Recent clinical trials indicate that retinoids may be used for prevention of cancers of the upper areas of the digestive tract, skin, breasts, and ovaries. Retinoids are potentially useful agents for cancer chemoprevention.[12] However, some studies actually point to a statistical association between high retinol levels and certain cancers and bring up the possibility that retinol may promote cancer development under some circumstances, especially when coupled with alcohol. Other reasons for the apparent association may be flawed or biased study designs and the fact that liver, the main dietary source of retinol in the United States, is also the most likely to concentrate environmental toxins.[13]

A study examining childhood and adult eating patterns found that the risks of cancer varied depending on age, weight, and diet. Postmenopausal women had a reduced risk of cancer if their diet had high levels of beta-carotene, specifically from carrots. In the same study, an association was found between girls having a heavier weight in childhood and adolescence and a lower risk of premenopausal breast cancer. Yet, heavier adult women increased their risk of postmenopausal breast cancer.[14]

Beta-carotene and retinol have also been found useful in treating women with premenopausal mastodynia.[15]

Many studies indicate that low levels of beta-carotene increase the risk of lung cancer.[16,17,18,19] Also, smokers who have a diet high in beta-carotene may be protected slightly more from the carcinogenic effects of smoking cigarettes than smokers with low beta-carotene levels.[20] Contradictory to these findings are the recently released results of the now famous Finnish smokers study published in April of 1994.[21] This randomized, double-blind trial followed smokers for five to eight years to see the effects of beta-carotene and vitamin E supplementation. Even the authors of the study were surprised to find that the beta-carotene group actually had a *higher* incidence of lung cancer than the placebo (inactive agent) group, leading to the uneasy conclusion that beta-carotene may actually be carcinogenic. No one has a ready explanation for these unexpected findings, considering that more than 100 previous epidemiologic studies have shown a link between high beta-carotene levels and reduced cancer risks. One of the most recent of these, which was also a double-blind, placebo-controlled study, was done in Linxian, China. It showed an overall reduction of 13 percent in cancer mortality.[22]

In another study, involving 1,271 subjects over 65 without cancer, it was found that future mortality from cancer appeared to be dependent on the consumption of foods high in beta-carotene. The individuals with low levels had the highest death rate due to cancer.[23]

In light of this conflict, everyone is waiting for the other shoe to drop, since several other large trials are currently under way.[24] All this being said, however, it appears obvious that nothing will dramatically reduce the risk of lung cancer but to quit smoking.

Topical and systemic derivatives of vitamin A, or retinoids, have been used successfully to treat acne and sun-damaged skin. (See Chapter 33 for further information.) Researchers are presently working on other vitamin A derivatives to help heal wounds and treat skin diseases such as psoriasis, actinic keratoses, and leukoplakia. A new study showed no beneficial effects were found regarding the prevention of nonmelanoma skin cancer with either retinol or isotrentinoin. The study consisted of the participants receiving either 10 milligrams of isotretinoin, a placebo, or 25,000 international units (IU) of retinol for a three-year period. There was no difference between the three groups.[25] Another study did conclude that retinol did reduce incidence of first new squamous cell skin cancers but had no effect on the incidence of first new basal cell skin cancer in moderate risk subjects.[26]

Food Sources of Beta-Carotene

Green leafy vegetables, carrots, broccoli, tomatoes, sweet potatoes, apricots, watermelon, cantaloupes, and papayas contain beta-carotene. The amount of the vitamin in the fruit or vegetable is dependent on the quality of the soil, amount of rainfall, and sunshine.[27]

Food Sources of Retinol

Retinol is found almost exclusively in animal products such as liver, kidney, milk, and fish. Fish liver oil is very high in retinol.

Recommendations

The RDA is 800 retinol equivalents (RE), or 4,000 IU, for adult women and pregnant women. The RDA for lactating (nursing) women is 1,300 RE, or 6,500 IU, for the first six months and 1,200 RE, or 6,000 IU, from six months on.

One study, conducted on 30 healthy men, examined the beta-carotene in foods and in supplements. It found that the plasma levels were higher in the individuals who consumed purified beta-carotene supplements rather than foods high in beta-carotene.[28]

Woman's Guide Suggestion

Supplement with 5,000 IU of vitamin A daily and 3 to 5 mg of beta-carotene daily.

Antagonists

Women who take estrogen may have a higher need for extra vitamin A. High estrogen intake has been shown to inhibit the absorption of the vitamin.[29] Oral contraceptives seem to reduce serum beta-carotene levels, especially for women over 35. Taking oral contraceptives appears to be an important risk factor causing higher vascular morbidity and mortality in women. It seems prudent to recommend a diet rich in beta-carotene especially for women taking oral contraceptives.[30]

Women who take large doses of vitamin E may need larger amounts of vitamin A since vitamin E inhibits absorption of vitamin A. Vitamin A is sensitive to acid and heat, and it oxidizes quickly on exposure to light and oxygen. Beta-carotene is also sensitive to heat.

Toxicity

Taken for extended periods, 15,000 to 25,000 IU of retinol per day may result in signs of vitamin A overdosage.[31, 32] Beta-carotene, at present, has not been shown to be toxic at any dose.

Warning

Vitamin A as retinol is poisonous in large amounts. Acute poisoning with massive doses can result in nausea, vomiting, headache, dizziness, abdominal pain, and even death. More common are cases of chronic poisoning, resulting in a wide range of symptoms, including dry, peeling skin, sore mouth, hair loss, brittle nails, dry eyes and blurred vision, decreased appetite, abdominal pain, weight loss, headache, fatigue, cramps, increased thirst, abnormal menses, arthritis, and liver abnormalities.[33] Patients admitted to psychiatric hospitals repeatedly for depression and schizophrenia have occasionally been shown to be suffering from hypervitaminosis A.[34]

Women who are pregnant or planning to become pregnant should not take more than 8,000 IU of vitamin A per day.[35] Birth defects have been associated with high levels of vitamin A intake, so check with a physician. Because of birth defects, oral retinoids for cystic acne are *absolutely contraindicated* in pregnant women or in women who may become pregnant during treatment.

4

The B Vitamins

Primary Functions

Maintains skin, hair, nails, eyes, and mucous membranes
Needed for nerve and brain function and memory
Necessary for liver function
Aids general metabolism
Maintains muscle tone
Required for blood cell production
Required for antibody production
Needed for production of sex hormones
Lowers cholesterol
Increases heat tolerance

The B vitamins, if used as a supplement, should be taken as a group in a B complex. The B vitamins work together, and a balance between them needs to be maintained. Consuming either too little or too much can cause problems. In many cases, a deficiency in one B vitamin may signal a deficiency in another. Check with a physician if you supplement with one particular B vitamin for a specific problem or deficiency.

There are 11 common B vitamins. They are all water-soluble and need to be replaced daily. The B vitamins consist of thiamine, riboflavin, niacin, pantothenic acid, pyridoxine (B_6), folic acid, cyanocobalamin (B_{12}), biotin, para-amino-benzoic acid (PABA), inositol, and choline. Three other compounds, occasionally touted as B vitamins—pangamic acid, orotic acid, and laetrile—are not commonly used in this country and are not considered essential vitamins.

Thiamine (B_1)

Thiamine keeps collagen-rich connective tissues and mucous membranes healthy and helps to maintain smooth muscle. It is known to help in the formation of the blood cells and is necessary for nervous system function. Low levels of thiamine can cause memory loss and mental deterioration. In a 1997 double-blind study, 120 young adult females with normal thiamine levels took either a placebo or 50 milligrams (mg) of thiamine each day for two months. The women's mood, memory, and reaction times were monitored. Those taking thiamine were more clearheaded, composed, and energetic than those in the control group, who showed decreased reaction times. But no effect on memory was shown.[1]

The classical deficiency disease, seen in people living on polished rice, is called *beriberi*. Two forms occur with weakness, confusion, and either swelling or wasting, depending on whether the primary tissue damage is heart or nerve tissue. Another result of thiaminee deficiency, *Wernicke-Korsakoff syndrome*, with nerve damage and memory loss, is seen occasionally in this country in alcoholics. Another study examined the effects of supplementation of thiaminee on male athletes who had either normal or low thiaminee levels. One hundred milligrams of thiaminee was given three days prior to exercising. The thiaminee significantly reduced the number of complaints of fatigue shortly after exercise. The reseachers did not know whether the thiaminee supplementation reduced fatigue or increased recovery time from fatigue.[2]

Food Sources of Thiamine

Whole grains and unmilled rice are high in thiamine as are beans and seafood.

Recommendations

The RDA for women aged 25 to 50 is 1.1 mg and from age 51 up is 1.0 mg. The RDA for pregnant women is 1.5 mg; for lactating women it is 1.6 mg.

Woman's Guide Suggestion

Supplement with 15 mg of thiamine daily.

Antagonists

Dieting and alcohol consumption are antagonists. Raw fish, coffee, tea, and betel nuts contain enzymes that destroy thiamine. The milling of rice and grains, cooking, and alkaline or acidic pH either inhibit or diminish the available thiamine. Folate deficiency decreases the absorption of thiamine.[3]

Toxicity

Thiamine can be ingested in large quantities without known problems, but large injected doses can rarely cause a reaction resembling *anaphylactic shock* (sudden collapse with respiratory distress and circulation failure).[4]

Riboflavin (B_2)

Riboflavin is necessary for healthy hair, nails, and mucous membranes. It is also important in red blood cell formation, antibody production, and overall growth.

Food Sources of Riboflavin

There are many foods that contain riboflavin including meat, eggs, legumes, fish, poultry, green, leafy vegetables, and fruits.

Recommendations

The RDA for women between the ages of 25 and 50 is 1.3 mg and for women 51 and older is 1.2 mg. The RDA for pregnant women is 1.6 mg; for lactating women in the first six months it is 1.8 mg and from six months on it is 1.7 mg.

Woman's Guide Suggestion

Supplement with 15 mg of riboflavin daily.

Antagonists

Sodium bicarbonate, an ingredient used to keep the green color in preserved vegetables, inhibits riboflavin absorption. Riboflavin is sensitive to light and to both acidic and alkaline environments. Also, soaking vegetables in water will leach out riboflavin.

Toxicity

There have been no reports of toxicity from riboflavin.

Warning

Women who exercise excessively or drink alcohol may need extra riboflavin. Women with *hypothyroidism* (low thyroid) are also at risk of having low levels of riboflavin.

Niacin (B_3)

Niacin is a generic name for a group of compounds that exhibit niacin activity. Nicotinic acid and niacinamide are most commonly used as supplements. Nicotinic acid comes from plants, and niacinamide comes from animal products. It is important to note that nicotinic acid but not niacinamide will raise *high-density lipoproteins* (HDLs). Nicotinic acid will cause a warm harmless flush that may be disturbing to some women. However, some authors claim that if an aspirin is taken prior to the niacin, the flushing will be reduced. Niacinamide does not evoke a flushing response. Another important chemical, *tryptophan*, is turned into niacin within the body. Tryptophan is found in both meats and vegetables.

In 1989 a problem appeared in some people taking l-tryptophan supplements, causing damage to nerves, brain, lung, muscle, and heart. This was apparently traced to a contaminant in the supplements produced by one manufacturer. Despite the fact that the disorder was traced to a contaminant and not l-tryptophan, the FDA pulled all l-tryptophan supplements off the market because of safety concerns.

Niacin helps in the production of most of the sex hormones. It dilates blood vessels, lowers cholesterol, and helps with overall circulation. Supplementation with 3 to 4 grams (g) per day of niacin elevates HDLs.[5,6] Further research has found that niacin at a dosage of 1 g per day helps reduce the incidence of recurrent myocardial infarction (heart attack).[7]

Severe, sustained niacin deficiency results in pellagra, marked by the "three Ds"—diarrhea, dementia, and dermatitis—and sometimes a fourth D, death. Pellegra used to be seen in the American Southwest among the Indian population which subsisted almost exclusively on corn, but now is seen mostly in inveterate alcoholics.

Food Sources of Niacin

Niacin is mostly found in meats, fish, and poultry.

Recommendations

The RDA for women ages 25 to 50 is 15 mg and for women 51 and up is 13 mg. The RDA for pregnant women is 17 mg; for lactating women it is 20 mg. For reducing bad cholesterol in high cholesterol patients, sustained-release niacin preparations were found to be more effective than the immediate-release type.[8]

Woman's Guide Suggestion

Under the age of 40, supplement with 30 mg of niacin daily; after the age of 40, supplement with 100 mg daily.

Toxicity

Nicotinic acid can cause various problems at levels of 3 to 9 g per day, including skin pigmentation and dryness, and, rarely, liver toxicity and elevated uric acid levels.[9]

Warning

Individuals with ulcers, liver disease, gout, or heart problems should consult a doctor before adding a supplement to the diet. Because of reported liver toxicity, periodic monitoring of liver enzymes may be advisable if you are taking sustained-release niacin.[10] Women who drink alcohol may need extra supplementation. Deficiencies of B6 and riboflavin will prevent tryptophan from being converted into niacin. Nicotinic acids enhance zinc and iron utilization. In vegetarian diets most of the niacin is in the bound form and therefore has low bioavailability.[11]

Pantothenic Acid (B_5)

Pantothenic acid has been used for a wide variety of reasons. It is important for the production of adrenal gland hormones and supposedly increases overall energy levels. It helps convert food into energy. It is found in almost all foods and is utilized in every tissue of the body. Pantothenic acid is known as the "antistress" vitamin.

Food Sources of Pantothenic Acid

B5 is found in whole wheat, beans, freshwater fish, meats, and fresh vegetables.

Recommendations

The RDA given for the safe and adequate intake for B5 is from 4 to 7 mg.

Woman's Guide Suggestion

Supplement with 25 mg of B5 daily.

Toxicity

Daily intake of 10 g per day of B5 has been reported to cause diarrhea and water retention.[12] Other toxic reactions are unknown.

Pyridoxine (B_6)

B6 actually refers to three different compounds: pyridoxine, pyridoxamine, and pyridoxal. B6 is probably involved in at least 100 different reactions in the body, from the production of RNA and DNA to relieving water retention. There are conflicting studies on the beneficial effect of high doses of B6 on premenstrual syndrome (PMS) symptoms. The Second National Health and Nutrition Examination Survey found that half the women surveyed had a B6 intake of less than 82 percent of the RDA for B6. A researcher, after trying a few different protocals, found that 100 mg of B6 daily corrected carpal tunnel syndrome over a 12-week period.[13] Crystalline pyridoxine hydrochloride is considered to be highly bioavailable.[14]

Food Sources of Pyridoxine

B6 is found in brewer's yeast, carrots, spinach, soybeans, eggs, chicken, walnuts, wheat germ, beans, saltwater fish, whole wheat, and fresh vegetables. Pyridoxine is found in plants, whereas pyridoxamine and pyridoxal are found in meats.

Recommendations

The RDA for women over 15 is 1.6 mg B6. The RDA for pregnant women is 2.2 mg; for lactating women it is 2.1 mg.

Woman's Guide Suggestion

Supplement with 50 mg of B6 daily.

Antagonists

Pyridoxine is light-sensitive, and pyridoxamine and pyridoxal are destroyed by high temperatures. Women who take estrogen or drink alcohol may need to supplement B_6.

Toxicity

There are problems associated with high doses of B_6. Chronic, large doses of B_6 in the 500 mg to 2 g per day range were reported to be neurotoxic in the early 1980s. Since then doses averaging 117 mg per day for a six-month period have been blamed for severe motor and sensory neuropathies.[15]

Warning

Alcohol, certain antituberculosis drugs, and drugs containing estrogen may increase the need for B_6. Women vegetarians and women who consume few animal products may have an increased need for B_6.

Folic Acid

Folic acid or folate is essential in the production of red blood cells, the production of hormones, and the synthesis of DNA.

Low serum folate levels are associated with an increased risk of fatal coronary heart disease. Folate is more bioavailable in supplements than it is from food.[16] Low folic acid levels may increase the risk of colon cancer. A 62 percent lower incidence of cancer was seen in patients with *chronic ulcerative colitis* (an inflammatory disease of the colon) who were given folic acid supplementation.[17] Folate supplementation may protect against the development of neoplasia in ulcerative colitis. Also, although there is no proof, evidence indicates that folic acid can also reduce the risk of dysplasia or colorectal cancer in patients with ulcerative colitis.[18]

Low levels of folic acid are associated with a birth defect known as *spina bifida*, in which the neural tube does not close completely during the first weeks of fetal development,[19] resulting in an open spine with variable degrees of paralysis and retardation. The U.S. Public Health Service recommends that women who might become pregnant take 0.4 mg of folic acid per day to reduce the risk of of the disorder.[20] However, a woman who has previously concieved a child with spina bifida should increase her supplementation to 4 mg per day if she might become pregnant.[21]

Dysplasia (abnormal cell growth, often seen on Pap smears) of the uterine cervix in women taking oral contraceptives has shown improvement with folic acid supplementation. Apparently a folic acid metabolic derangement may be wrongly diagnosed as cervical dysplasia. The problem has been shown to be arrested or reversed with oral folic acid supplementation.[22] However, a later study by some of the same investigators failed to demonstrate the same effect.[23] Various studies have shown that red blood cell folate level is a good predictor of cervical dysplasia, although it may be protective against ***human papilloma***, or wart, ***virus*** (HPV) rather than dysplasia itself.[24] HPV, human papillomavirus, has been identified as the central cause for increased risk of cervical neoplasia. Also, low vitamin C and carotenoid status are also associated with cervical cancer and its precursors. Any effects of folate status may be restricted to early preneoplastic cervical lesions and not to a more advanced disease.[25]

Recent research suggests that supplementation with folate may help some memory and emotional disorders in older people, but so far no controlled studies have been done for confirmation.[26]

Food Sources of Folic Acid

The highest amounts of folate are found in liver and other organ meats, some fruits, legumes, yeast, and fresh greens.

Recommendations

The RDA is 180 micrograms (mcg) per day for women aged 25 and up. The RDA for pregnant women is 400 mcg. The RDA for lactating women in the first six months is 280 mcg and drops to 260 mcg from six months on.

It was reported that a daily folate intake of 200 to 250 mcg meets the needs of nonpregnant women. However, 300 mcg of folate per day allows room for a little extra storage.[27]

Folate deficiency is common in pregnant women in specific populations.[28] Folic acid supplements given before pregnancy have been shown to reduce the incidence of neural tube defects in newborns.[29]

Woman's Guide Suggestion

Supplement with 400 mcg of folic acid daily.

Antagonists

Alcohol interferes with folate utilization. Up to 95 percent of folate can be destroyed by cooking, refining, and canning. Folic acid and some anticonvulsant drugs inhibit each other's absorption. Oral contraceptives increase folate excretion in the urine. This may be responsible for the reduced serum and red cell folate levels seen in oral contraceptive users.[30]

Toxicity

Very high levels of supplemental folic acid (100 times the RDA) may precipitate convulsions in an epileptic patient on phenytoin by interfering with absorption of the seizure medicine. No significant problems were seen in a study giving women 10 mg folate daily for four months. However, folic acid supplementation of 400 mcg per day has been shown to interfere with zinc absorption.[31]

Warnings

Folic acid can mask a B_{12} deficiency, resulting in brain damage. Check with a physician before increasing folic acid consumption. Women who use oral contraceptives have a higher urinary loss of folate.

Cyanocobalamin (B_{12})

B_{12} is necessary for overall metabolism and nervous system function. It is also essential for the metabolism of folic acid. B_{12} is needed to make red blood cells and therefore is necessary to prevent *anemia*. Complaints of a B_{12} deficiency include nerve dysfunction, spasticity, confusion, dementia, and visual loss. B_{12} deficiencies occur in strict vegetarians, older people with loss of stomach acid, and in persons with *pernicious anemia* (a previously fatal illness due to an inability to absorb B_{12}). The deficiency can take 3 to 15 years to develop since the body is so conservative with its stores. A Dutch study in 1995 concluded that although B_{12} deficiency causes dementia, it is not a common cause of reversible dementia.[32] B_{12} must always be added to any folate fortification or supplementation.[33]

Food Sources of Vitamin B_{12}

B_{12} is not found in vegetables except some seaweeds and fermented soy products such as tofu. In these exceptions, the B_{12} is actually produced by bacteria rather than being intrinsic in the vegetable sources. It is mostly found in meats such as beef and pork. Vegetarians often have a deficiency.

Recommendations

The RDA for females aged 14 and up is 2.0 mcg. The RDA for pregnant women is 2.2 mcg; for lactating women it is 2.6 mcg.

Woman's Guide Suggestion

Supplement with 50 mcg of B_{12} daily.

Antagonists

Alcohol and medications for gout may interfere with the absorption of B_{12}.

Toxicity

No known toxic level exists.

Biotin

Biotin is necessary for the metabolism of carbohydrates, proteins, and fats. It is needed for healthy hair and skin. Some say that it will prevent hair from turning gray, although there is little research to support this.

Food Sources of Biotin

Biotin is found in salt-water fish, cooked egg yolks, soybeans, poultry, milk, whole grains, and yeast.

Recommendations

The RDA for the safe and adequate intake of biotin is 30 to 100 mcg.

Woman's Guide Suggestion

Supplement with 50 mcg of biotin daily.

Antagonists

Sulfa drugs, antibiotics, and raw egg whites inhibit the absorption of biotin.

Toxicity

No known toxic levels exist.

Para-Aminobenzoic Acid (PABA)

It has been claimed, yet not substantiated, that PABA restores gray hair to its original color. It does aid in the metabolization of proteins and in the production of red blood cells. PABA applied topically acts as a sunscreen and blocks out the dangerous ultraviolet B rays.

Food Sources of PABA

PABA is found in molasses, whole grains, kidney, and liver.

Recommendations

No RDA is listed for PABA.

Woman's Guide Suggestion

Supplement with 30 mg of PABA daily.

Antagonists

Sulfa drugs, alcohol, and estrogen may inhibit the absorption of PABA and cause a deficiency.

Warning

Allergic rashes to topical PABA sunscreens are relatively common.

Inositol

Inositol is essential for healthy hair. It helps remove fats from the arteries and the liver. It has been noted to be necessary for brain function.

Food Sources of Inositol

Inositol can be found in fruit, meat, milk, and whole grains.

Recommendations

No RDA is listed for inositol.

Woman's Guide Suggestion

Supplement with 80 mg of inositol daily.

Antagonists

Milling removes most of the inositol in grains. Caffeine, alcohol, and estrogen inhibit inositol absorption.

Choline

Choline is necessary for nervous system and brain function. A deficiency may cause memory problems. It is also important for gallbladder and liver function.[34] Large amounts of choline can be supplied as lecithin (phosphatidylcholine), a commonly used choline supplement and food additive. Lecithin, polyunsaturated fatty acids, vitamin C, and other B vitamins have been shown to reduce the risk of atherosclerosis. (See Chapter 5.)

Food Sources of Choline

Egg yolks, meat, milk, whole grains, and soybeans are high in choline.

Recommendations

The National Research Council has not determined whether choline is a necessary nutrient. However, the American Academy of Pediatrics has recommended that 7 mg be contained in 100 calories of baby formula, which is the same percentage found in human breast milk.[35]

Woman's Guide Suggestion

Supplement with 50 mg of choline daily.

Toxicity

Large doses can cause gastrointestinal distress, vomiting, sweating, salivation, and a fishy body odor.[36]

5

Vitamin C

PRIMARY FUNCTIONS

Necessary for the synthesis of collagen
Fights infection, reduces inflammation, and heals wounds
Acts as antioxidant
Reduces risk of heart disease
Lowers cholesterol
Reduces risk of lung, stomach, and esophageal cancers
Reduces cervical epithelial abnormalities (as reflected by Pap smears)
Inhibits N-nitrosamine (a carcinogen or cancer-causing agent)
Reduces the severity of colds

VITAMIN C IS necessary for the synthesis of *collagen*,[1] a major component of bone, skin, blood vessels, and muscles. A deficiency of vitamin C will inhibit new growth and compromise the health of these tissues. Adequate vitamin C is also critical for healthy gums, and bleeding gums are one of the first signs of a significant vitamin C deficiency. Ehlers-Danlos syndrome, a disease of impaired collagen production, has shown marked improvement after prolonged treatment with vitamin

C.[2] Also, vitamin C is regularly given to patients with skin ulcers to increase healing and shorten healing time.[3]

Vitamin C helps build the immune system and assists in fighting infection. It has been suggested that vitamin C reduces and modulates inflammation because of its antioxidant abilities.[4,5,6] Vitamin C may be the most important water-phase antioxidant for protection against diseases and degenerative processes caused by oxidative stress to the body.[7]

From 1971 to 1974, the National Health and Nutrition Study (known as NHANES I) sampled 11,348 people between the ages of 25 and 74.[8] The Epidemiologic Study (known as NHEFS) was a follow-up study on these same people in 1984. During the ten-year period, there were 1,809 deaths. Examination of the causes of death indicated that the people who had low levels of vitamin C had higher mortality rates and more deaths due to heart disease and cancer than did people who supplemented their diets with vitamin C. The amount of vitamin C necessary for the increased health benefits was a dietary consumption of 50 mg a day *plus* daily vitamin C supplementation.[9] Higher mortality was attributed more to low dietary levels of vitamin C than to high dietary levels of cholesterol or fat.[10]

Seven hundred female nurses who participated in the Nurses Health Study filled out a dietary questionnaire including all known and suspected risk factors for cancer and heart disease. The results indicated that the long-term (10 years or more), consumption of vitamin C supplements substantially reduced the development of age-related lens opacities by 77 percent. It is not known whether short-term supplementation is effective.[11]

Another study, that researched hundreds of males from different industrialized countries, found that many of the men had low plasma levels of vitamin C. A correlation between low plasma vitamin C levels and a higher risk of heart disease was found.[12] There is evidence that vitamin C has a protective effect against stroke, whereas there is less evidence that it is protective against coronary heart disease. This was based on a Medline search from articles written from 1980 to 1996.[13,14] Vitamin C offers protection against raised blood pressure and strokes.[15] Another study assessed the nutritional status of 747 Massachusetts people over a 9- to 12-year period. The results indicated that the individuals who consumed high intakes, over 400 mg per day, of vitamin C through vegetables were protected more against early mortality and mortality from heart disease than people who consumed less than 90 mg per day. However, this was not true for individuals who just used supplements and did not consume a diet high in vegetables.[16] This evidence does lead to the suspicion that vitamin C may be an indicator of the other beneficial nutrients or may need cofactors found in foods for optimal preformance.

Vitamin C has been shown to reduce cholesterol levels in a study of 50 subjects taking 2 g of vitamin C per day for a two-month period. Cholesterol and triglyceride levels decreased significantly, whereas HDLs increased.[17] Other researchers have concluded that in order to reduce atherosclerosis the diet needs to be supplemented not only with vitamin C but also with B_6 in a B complex, polyunsaturated fatty acids, and lecithin.[18] (See Chapter 4.)

Cancer is the second leading cause of death in the United States. Some authorities suspect that a majority of cases may be related to environmental factors. The antioxidant vitamins have been correlated with reduced risks of many cancers, and vitamin C has been associated with reduction in the risk of stomach and esophageal cancers in particular.[19] Among the known cancer-causing factors are *N-nitroso compounds*. These are found in cured meats and fish, alcoholic drinks, tobacco, and cigarette smoke and are also produced in the body's gastrointestinal tract. Vitamin C inhibits the formation and absorption of N-nitrosamines,[20] but not until the dietary intake of vitamin C reaches 1,000 mg per day.

Low plasma levels of vitamin C in cigarette smokers may exacerbate smoking-related lung damage since vitamin C has been shown to neutralize harmful oxidants produced in smokers' lungs.[21] Vitamin C appears to protect against deterioration of pulmonary function.[22]

Studies of otherwise healthy women with false-positive readings on their *Papanicolaou* (Pap) tests revealed that a significant number of the women had low plasma levels of vitamin C. The authors of this study suggested a possible relationship between low levels of vitamin C and the possibility of the occurance of cervical cancer in the future. Further research was suggested.[23]

A few years ago vitamin C was touted as the cure for the common cold. The more ambitious claims did not hold up to later research. However, convincing evidence exists that a higher level of vitamin C will indeed lessen the severity and shorten the length of a cold, even if it does not entirely prevent it.[24,25,26] Experiments on vitamin C carried out since the early 1970s have consistently shown that vitamin C supplementation alleviates the symptoms of the common cold. In most of the studies reviewed, the individuals took 1 to 3 g of vitamin C a day. The studies that found vitamin C to be ineffective had flawed methodology.[27]

Vitamin C has shown to lessen the risk of cartilage loss and disease progression in people with osteoarthritis of the knee, according to data collated after reviewing 640 participants' dietary intakes. Progression of osteoporosis and the development of knee pain seems to be reduced in people with high intakes of vitamin C. However, there was no evidence that increased vitamin C protects against the incidence of knee osteoarthritis.[28]

Bioflavonoids, also known as vitamin P, consist of hundreds of chemical compounds found in plants. Bioflavonoids are essential to the absorption of vitamin C. They also have estrogenic effects. They have 1/50,000 the activity of estrogen. Bioflavonoids have been shown to reduce bleeding, improve vaginal lubrication, strengthen the bladder, reduce water retention, ease sore joints, decrease or end hot flashes, improve liver activity, reduce muscle cramping, strengthen resistance to infections, and possibly lower the risk of stroke and heart disease.[29]

Bioflavonoids, rutin, and hesperidin are relatively common ingredients in vitamin supplements. Bioflavonoids are found in the white part of citrus fruit, in rosehips, apricots, cherries, green peppers, tomatoes, and blackberries. Proanthocyanidins are a group of polyphenolic bioflavonoids. They have been reported to exhibit chemoprotective properties against oxygen free radicals. Included in this group are grape seed extract, vitamin C, and vitamin E succinate. However, grape seed extract was found to be a better oxygen free radical scavenger than C or E.[30]

Just recently the media has made an unjustified splash about vitamin C being a potentially harmful pro-oxidant. A 1998 British in vivo study showed that vitamin C, at a dose of 500 mg per day, can cause oxidative *damage* to adenine bases in the chromosomal DNA material of human lymphocytes, producing 8-oxoadenine. The study also showed that vitamin C provided an equal degree of oxidative *protec-*

tion to another DNA base, preventing guanine from oxidizing to 8-oxoguanine.[31] On its surface this appears to be an even trade. However, it turns out that damage to guanine bases is about 10 times as likely to result in mutations as is damage to adenine bases, so the data may actually be interpreted as quite favorable to vitamin C rather than critical. Considering this, the authors were surprised at the anti-vitamin C spin given the article by the news media.[32]

Food Sources of Vitamin C

Sources include broccoli, green peppers, tomatoes, cabbages, oranges, green, leafy vegetables, strawberries, and grapefruit. Small amounts of vitamin C are also found in milk, meats, and cereal.

Recommendations

The RDA for females 15 years and older is 60 mg. The RDA for pregnant women is 70 mg. The RDA for lactating women in the first six months is 95 mg and 90 mg from six months on. Recommendations by various groups around the world vary from 30 mg to 120 mg per day. Dr. Pauling, a well-known but controversial researcher, is quoted as recommending 2.3 to 9.5 g of vitamin C per day.[33]

Woman's Guide Suggestion

Supplement with 500 to 1,500 mg (500 mg three times per day) of vitamin C daily. Also, supplement with 100 mg of bioflavonoids daily.

Antagonists

Vitamin C is destroyed by heat, light, oxidation on exposure to air, prolonged storage, and alkali. Women who use oral contraceptives, take any form of estrogen, are pregnant or lactating, smoke, drink alcohol, or have undergone surgery may need extra vitamin C in their diets. Nonsteroidal anti-inflammatory drugs such as ibuprofen, corticosteroids, and antibiotics may also deplete vitamin C.[34]

Toxicity:

The toxicity levels of vitamin C are unknown. Higher dosages will cause diarrhea.

Warning

High doses can cause false readings on some medical tests such as guaiac tests for blood in the stool and tests for sugar in the urine. Kidney stones and gout have been attributed to a high consumption of vitamin C. However, even at high levels, vitamin C does not cause or worsen kidney stones unless the individual is predisposed to them or already has them.[35] It has been reported that abruptly discontinuing large doses of vitamin C can cause rebound scurvy in mothers and their newborn babies, but these reports are poorly documented.[36] Chewable vitamin C can cause damage to the enamel on teeth. Vitamin C increases the absorption of iron. This may not be a problem in premenopausal years, but may cause some problems after menopause. (See Chapter 16.)

6

Vitamin D

Primary Functions

Aids mineralization and calcification of bone
Prevents rickets in children
Prevents osteomalacia (bone softening) in adults
Aids bone and tooth preservation and growth
May lower blood pressure

Vitamin D, a fat soluble vitamin, is both a hormone and a vitamin. With help from the sun's rays, it can be produced in the skin from a cholesterol compound and can also be absorbed from foods in the diet. Vitamin D must be metabolized by the liver and kidney before it is active.

Vitamin D is partly responsible for bone calcification and bone mineralization. Low levels of vitamin D can cause rickets in children and osteomalacia in older people. Both conditions are abnormalities of bone mineralization resulting in soft bones. The bioavailability of calcium is increased when vitamin D is added to a supplement. Research suggests that calcium carbonate with vitamin D given three times daily, twice at meals and once at bedtime, is the best regime for absorption of calcium.[1] (See Chapter 24.)

Bone loss speeds up around the menopause. Sometimes women begin to lose bone density even before they actually stop menstruating.[2] Vitamin D is critical in helping to preserve bones and teeth in perimenopausal women, and supplementation has been shown to retard bone loss during this time.[3] As women age, vitamin D absorption slows down. This compounds a problem since the skin no longer synthesizes vitamin D as efficiently, and the liver and kidney conversion of vitamin D declines. An intake of 400 to 800 IU per day will maintain in elderly people the same blood levels of vitamin D that are considered normal in young people.[4] These levels of supplementation are considered safe over long periods.[5]

Bone loss is apparently seasonal,[6] as are vitamin D levels. Most people get sufficient vitamin D from natural sun exposure, adequate sunshine being approximately 15 minutes per day. This is a problem for people who live in cloudy areas or at high latitudes, as demonstrated by the higher rate of osteomalacia in Great Britain than in sunnier locations. There also tends to be more bone loss during cloudy months than during sunny ones. One hypothesis is that decreased vitamin D causes a rise in parathyroid hormone levels during winter, in turn causing an increase in bone turnover. A study of 333 women living in Massachusetts found that women who took more than 220 IU of vitamin D per day maintained a constant parathyroid hormone level throughout the year rather than having seasonal changes.[7] Women in Canada have been found to have low levels of vitamin D and are advised to supplement their diets.[8]

Low levels of vitamin D and calcium have also been associated with increased blood pressure in older women.[9]

Recently the FDA approved a new vitamin D analog cream for the topical treatment of psoriasis.

Food Sources of Vitamin D

Vitamin D is found in fatty salt water fish, milk products, egg yolks, and liver. There is some concern that the current trends in "eating smart" i. e., cutting back on fatty, high-cholesterol, high-calorie foods inadvertently may substantially lower the vitamin D intake in some persons. A theoretical concern also exists about the possibility that the recent widespread use of sunscreens may significantly interfere with vitamin D production in the skin in people with marginal dietary intake of vitamin D.

Recommendations

The RDA for women 25 and over is 200 IU. The RDA for women who are pregnant or lactating is 400 IU per day.

Woman's Guide Suggestion

Supplement with 400 IU of vitamin D daily.

Antagonists

Anticonvulsant therapy and some liver and kidney diseases can block the positive effects of vitamin D. Sun-damaged skin and darkly pigmented skin slow down vitamin D synthesis from ultraviolet rays, as do sunscreens.

Toxicity

1,000 to 1,800 IU of vitamin D per day can cause severe problems, especially in young children. These problems include soft tissue calcification with heart and kidney damage. On the other hand, an elderly patient with senile osteoporosis (bone thinning with easy fractures) can often take up to 100,000 IU per day without toxicity.[10]

7

Vitamin E

Primary Functions

Acts as antioxidant
Needed for maintenance of cell membranes
Needed for neurological health
May relieve hot flashes
May relieve mastodynia or sore breasts
May help fibrocystic breast disease
May reduce incidence of mammary tumors
May relieve PMS symptoms
Works synergistically with selenium and CoQ10
May reduce the risk of lung cancer
May reduce the risk of heart disease
May slow progression of Alzheimer's disease

VITAMIN E, A fat-soluble vitamin, is the generic name for a technical group of eight compounds: four tocopherols—alpha, beta, gamma, and delta—and four tocotrenols. Alpha-tocopherol is the most active form of vitamin E.

Vitamin E, commonly known as an antioxidant, protects polyunsaturated fats from spoiling or oxidizing. It does this effectively in cell membranes and is one of the major agents that keep cell membranes healthy. Evidence also shows that vitamin E has an important role maintaining neurological health. Some researchers recommend that individuals who have fat malabsorption problems or vitamin E deficiencies supplement their diets with vitamin E in order to avoid neurological abnormalities.[1]

Many individuals have claimed that vitamin E relieves hot flashes associated with menopause. Although this has not been successfully documented in the scientific medical research, many women affirm its efficacy after supplementing their diets with vitamin E. Vitamin E is reported to limit the excessive menopausal production of follicle-stimulating and luteinizing hormones (FSH and LH) respectively.[2] Based on anecdotal information, one author suggested that vitamin E in the recommended doses may work and will not cause harm.[3] Perry and O'Hanlan, in *Natural Menopause*, state that nutritionists' recommendations of 1000 mg of vitamin E, 500 mg of vitamin C, and a B-complex vitamin, with or without 25 mcg of selenium may provide relief.[4] Ruth Jacobowitz, the author of *150 Most-Asked Questions about Menopause*, states that she personally took 400 mg of vitamin E twice daily, with relief of her symptoms.[5]

Breast soreness, or mastodynia, is a complaint of many women. It can be attributed to a number of different causes, most of which are not serious. However, in some cases mastodynia may be a symptom of more dire problems such as breast cancer. In the book *Menopause and the Years Ahead*, the authors suggested that when mastodynia results from estrogen or hormone replacement therapy (ERT/HRT), women should try vitamin E along with ibuprofen and the elimination of all caffeine, *for a week or so only*, to see if the symptoms subside.[6]

Fibrocystic breast disease increases with premenopausal age and decreases after menopause. It is aggravated by high levels of estrogen and low levels of progesterone. The symptoms of the disease include breast tenderness, nodularity, fibrocystic plaques, macrocysts, and fibrocystic lumps. This disease may increase a woman's risk of future breast cancer. Fibrocystic breast disease has been treated with estrogen and progestins, or progestins alone to counter the estrogens. These treatments have also been used in conjunction with vitamin E supplementation. In very mild cases of the disorder, vitamin E alone has been shown to alleviate some of the problems.[7] However, in several double-blind studies, other researchers concluded that treating fibrocystic breast disease with vitamin E was without benefit.[8, 9, 10]

One review of the literature proposed that supplementation of vitamin E at higher levels than the recommended dietary allowances may reduce the future risk of breast cancer. It was noted that vitamin E helped reduce the incidence of mammary tumors. Whether vitamin E worked as a cellular antioxidant or as an agent that improves DNA replication or both was unknown, and the authors suggested that large scale research be conducted.[11]

Another group came to a different conclusion when they examined 120 women with breast cancer and compared them with 109 women in a control group. The group found higher serum levels of vitamin E and a reduced level of lipid peroxidation in the breast cancer population. (Lipid peroxidation is low in rapidly proliferating tissues such as cancers.) It is suspected that vitamin E is a factor in reducing peroxidation levels. This study concluded that high levels of vitamin E are associated with an *increased* risk of premenopausal breast cancer, but that the high vitamin E levels may be the result rather than the cause of the cancers or may be coincidental.[12]

Another study concluded that since vitamin E protects cells from oxidant damage, vitamin E may protect breast tissue from such damage that may lead to the development of cancer. The researchers concluded that dietary supplementation of vitamin E in excess of dietary RDA requirement may reduce the women's risk of developing breast cancer.[13]

A randomized double-blind study on 41 women with PMS found that treating the women with 400 IU of alpha-tocopherol daily reduced their symptoms. The women found improvement in specific affective and physical complaints.[14]

Selenium and vitamin E have a synergistic relationship. Selenium is needed for the functioning of the antioxidant enzyme glutathione peroxidase, which also protects membrane lipids, and the two need each other to work properly in the body. Presently, there is concern, because of poorer soil conditions, that our diets may be deficient in selenium.[15] (See Chapter 21.) In a mineral- and vitamin-deficient area of China in Linxian province, a double-blind study was recently completed. Subjects supplemented with a combination of vitamin E, selenium, and beta-carotene showed a reduction of cancer deaths by 13 percent.[16]

Research was conducted on 99 people who had lung cancer compared with 196 normal controls in Washington County, Maryland. The researchers studied the relationships between serum beta-carotene, retinol, vitamin E, and the risk of lung cancer. The results of the study indicated that low serum levels of vitamin E were associated with increased risk of all types of lung cancer and low levels of beta-carotene were associated with increased risk of squamous-cell carcinoma of the lung specifically.[17]

Vitamin E supplementation may increase the rate of rebuilding muscles after exercising, especially in older individuals.[18] Evidence also exists that vitamin E may be helpful when exercising in high altitudes.[19] Human studies on exercise support dietary supplementation of antioxidant vitamins. They have favorable effects on lipid peroxidation after exercise and protect against exercise-induced muscle damage. Free radical production increases during exercise. Vitamin E is consumed by muscles and other tissues during increased physical activity.[20] (See Chapter 27.)

A heart disease study of adherence patterns of blood platelets in healthy men and women found that platelets preferred to adhere to places that had been previously occupied by blood clots. In addition to this, there was a remarkable decrease in platelet adherence observed after vitamin E supplementation. Vitamin E was given as d-alpha-tocopherol over a four-week period: 200 IU were given for two weeks and 400 IU were given the second two weeks. The average decrease in adhesion after two weeks was 75 percent and after four weeks was 82 percent.[21] This may protect against heart disease by discouraging blood clots.

In the Cambridge Heart Antioxidant Study (CHAOS), 2,002 patients with confirmed coronary artery disease were given either a placebo or vitamin E, either 400 IU or 800 IU per day for approximately 510 days. The study showed the group of patients who consumed 400 IU of vitamin E per day had reduced nonfatal myocardial infarctions by 77 percent. However, the death rates from cardiovascular disease were not reduced.[22] In the MONICA/WHO cross-cultural comparison of 16 European populations and the very large health professionals' studies, vi-tamin E was consistently associated with lowered risk of disease.[23]

Three other large studies found that individuals who supplemented with vitamin E had approximately 40 percent lower rates of coronary heart disease than nonusers. Both 400 and 800 IU of vitamin E per day showed a strong reduction in nonfatal myocardial infarction, whereas 100 IU had no effect.[24] The Cambridge Heart Antioxidant Study found vitamin E, alpha tocopherol, to be the most promising antioxidants for the lessening of heart disease. Supplementation of vitamin E after four days had a positive effect on LDL. However, 14 days after stopping the supplement the benefits diminished.[25] In the Nurses Health Study, which consisted of 87,000 nurses, the women who consumed more than 100 IU of vitamin E per day for two years had a significant reduction in nonfatal myocardial infarction and reduced mortality from cardiovascular disease by approximately 30 percent.[26] Supplementation with vitamin E seems like a logical intervention strategy to prevent coronary heart disease.[27, 28, 29]

In 1997 a study made the media headlines, claiming that 800 IU of vitamin E and 1 g of vitamin C given before a fatty meal will reduce the "bad" cornary effects of the fatty meal. The study did support this claim but the purpose of the study was to demonstrate the oxidative effects of the vitamins, not to suggest that it be used as a protective element for eating "bad" foods.[30]

CoQ10 works synergistically with vitamin E. Studies indicated that the combination may reduce the risk of both heart disease and cancer. (See Chapter 9.)

A statistically lower level of alpha-tocopherol was observed in the blood serum of human papillomavirus-infected women with cervical dysplasia. The risk of dysplasia was four times higher when the levels were less than 7.95 umol/l. Vitamin E blood levels might be useful as a bio marker of the risk of dysplasia in the infected women.[31]

In a double-blind study of 341 patients with severe Alzheimer's disease, vitamin E and/or selegiline slowed the progression of the disease when compared to the placebo group. One quarter of the patients was given 2,000 IU of vitamin E and selegiline per day, the second quarter was given just 2,000 IU of vitamin E, the third quarter was given selegiline, and the fourth quarter was given a placebo over a two-year period.[32]

Food Sources of Vitamin E

Sources include wheat germ oil, corn oil, safflower oil, soybean oil, wheat germ, mango, lettuce, green peas, brown rice, egg yolk, liver, nuts, vegetables, cereal grains, sesame seeds, liver, haddock, mackerel, and herring.

This list of sources, although technically accurate, may not be useful in a practical sense. This is because the required amount of vitamin E necessary daily is dependent on the amount of polyunsaturated fatty acids (PUFA) consumed in the diet. Vitamin E protects PUFA from peroxidation. So, as the levels of PUFA increase, so do necessary levels of vitamin E. PUFA also slows the absorption of vitamin E.[33] High levels of PUFA can actually cause a vitamin E deficiency if the diet is marginal in vitamin E. For example, a walnut is high in vitamin E, and it is very high in PUFA. Protecting the large amount of PUFA in walnuts from peroxidation requires more vitamin E than walnuts contain. Wheat germ oil is an excellent source of vitamin E, containing 215 mg per 100 g of oil and needing only 41 mg for oxidative protection. But corn oil is a net wash, needing all of its vitamin E for its own oxidative protection. And safflower oil, widely touted as a vitamin E source, actually uses up 11 mg more of vitamin E than 100 g of oil contain. This is why people who eat large amounts of polyunsaturated fats need to increase their vitamin E intake.

Large amounts of fish liver oils, commonly used as a vitamin A supplement, also increase the need for vitamin E.

Recommendations

The RDA for adult women 25 and above is 8 mg. The recommended level for pregnant women is 10 mg. The RDA for lactating women in months one to six is 12 mg and after six months is 11 mg. An intake of 200 to 800 mg, which is 20 to 80 times the suggested levels, has been considered safe.[34]

Woman's Guide Suggestion

Supplement with 400 to 800 mg of vitamin E daily.

Antagonists

Vitamin E is quite unstable. Both cooking and storage reduce availability of the vitamin. Estrogen and high levels of iron may interfere with vitamin E absorption. Therefore, inorganic iron or birth control pills should be taken separately from vitamin E.[35]

Toxicity

A review has indicated that a person would have to take up to 3,200 IU per day before any consistent side effects would be seen.[36]

Warning

Vitamin E can produce coagulation problems if there is a vitamin K deficiency.[37] Large doses of vitamin E may increase the need for vitamin K and may result in bleeding problems in persons taking blood thinners.[38] Vitamin E has a mild antiplatelet effect. It should be discontinued prior to any planned surgical procedures. Check with your physician.[39]

8

Vitamin K

Primary Functions

Needed for blood clotting
Helps growth of bones

Vitamin K is needed for normal blood clotting. In fact, blood thinners such as Coumadin work by inhibiting the action of vitamin K. Signs of deficiency are easy bruising, slow clotting, and bleeding gums. However, except in cases of severe intestinal malabsorption, kidney failure, or antibiotic therapy in debilitated patients, vitamin K-related bleeding problems are rare in adults. The amount of vitamin K contained in the diet and synthesized in the intestines is otherwise sufficient to prevent bleeding abnormalities.

Actions of vitamin K concerning bone maintenance are probably more germane to the concerns of healthy adult women. Research on vitamin K's role in bone formation has been ongoing, if not continuous, over the past 20 years. A few studies have shown that supplementation with vitamin K reduces calcium loss in postmenopausal women.[1,2] A 1984 study, done on osteoporotic patients with either spinal crush fractures or femoral neck fractures, determined that the circulating vitamin K levels were as much as one-third lower than in individuals without osteoporosis.[3] A recent study in 1991 suggested that serum levels of vitamin K may be useful as a tool to predict osteoporosis.[4] Another study in 1997 supported the earlier findings. The levels of vitamin K were measured in 71 postmenopausal women, 19 with reduced bone mineral density and 52 with normal bone density. The women with reduced bone mineral density showed lower levels of vitamin K_1 and K_2 than those with normal bone density.[5] More long-term research is needed to further elucidate the role of vitamin K in bone growth and the necessary dietary requirements for humans.[6,7]

Taking this hypothesis one step further, a study found an association between the presence of atherosclerotic calcifications in postmenopausal women, low bone mass, and an impaired vitamin K status.[8]

Vitamin K_1, known as phylloquinone, is found in plants and must be ingested. K_2, known as menaquinone, is produced in the gut by intestinal bacteria. K_2 is also found in some animal tissues. Vitamin K_3, known as menadione, is the synthetic form that can be converted by the liver to menaquinone. It has been alleged that vitamin K_2 may be more biologically active than K_1.[9] Many of the K vitamins presently sold on the market are in the form of K_1.

Food Sources of Vitamin K

Vitamin K is found in some green, leafy vegetables, broccoli, cauliflower, spinach, brussels sprouts, soybeans, coffee, green tea, butter, liver, bacon.

Recommendations

The National Academy of Sciences first gave a recommendation for a dietary allowance of vitamin K in 1989. The RDA for women is 65 mcg. No special allowance was made for pregnant or lactating women. *Most multivitamins do not contain vitamin K.*

Yogurt and kefir (with lactobacillus) keep the bacteria levels high in the intestines, resulting in adequate vitamin K synthesis.[10]

Woman's Guide Suggestion

Supplement with 10 mcg of vitamin K daily.

Antagonists

Androgens enhance a deficiency of vitamin K. Estrogen acts as a protector.[11] Absorption is inhibited by large doses of vitamin E, mineral oil, laxatives, and prolonged intravenous feeding. When given to pregnant mothers, anticonvulsants can block vitamin K and cause serious hypoprothrombinemia (a blood clotting factor deficiency) in newborns. Antibiotic therapy or intestinal disorders that cause problems with fat absorption can antagonize the absorption of vitamin K. Vitamin K deficiencies are not common in adults yet are quite common in newborn children. Vitamin K does not pass through the placenta very well, and babies' intestines are sterile at birth.

Toxicity

Toxic manifestations of vitamin K are unknown except when given as menadione in massive doses to newborns.[12, 13]

Warning

Do not take vitamin K while taking a blood thinner such as Coumadin without a physician's approval.

9

CoQ_{10}

Primary Functions

Reduces risk of heart disease
May protect against cancer
Increases physical performance

CoQ_{10} IS ALSO known as coenzyme Q_{10}, vitamin Q, and ubiquinone. The names are interchangeable. CoQ_{10} is biosynthesized from the amino acid tyrosine in a complicated process requiring each of eight different vitamins: tetrahydrobiopterin, B_2, B_6, C, B_{12}, niacin, pantothenic acid, and folic acid.[1]

CoQ_{10} works as an antioxidant with vitamin E synergistically to prevent early oxidation of low density lipoprotein (LDL), which is thought to be a first step in the development of atherosclerotic plaques. Supplementation with vitamin E alone results in LDL that is more prone to initial oxidation. When CoQ_{10} is added, it prevents the pro-oxidant activity of vitamin E and provides the lipoprotein with increased resistance to oxidation. There is reason to think that CoQ_{10} can protect against arteriosclerosis, and supplementation may be warranted for this reason alone.[2,3] Ironically, some of the drugs used for lowering cholesterol also interfere with the synthesis of CoQ_{10} and reduce CoQ_{10} levels, too. This could well decrease heart and liver function as well as being counterproductive in the prevention of arteriosclerosis unless CoQ10 is added to the diet.[4, 5]

CoQ10 is a busy molecule. Every cell in the body needs it for the production of ATP, the chemical energy that cells run on. Tissues with very high energy requirements have (or need) very high levels of CoQ10. The heart especially has a great need for CoQ10, and heart failure is correlated with decreasing tissue and blood levels of the molecule.[6]

Study after study, many of them placebo-controlled, have shown CoQ10 to increase the efficiency of the heart muscle's performance. It is used commonly as an adjunct to other cardiac and blood pressure medicines in the treatment of congestive heart failure and cardiomyopathy.[7, 8] Its use in the treatment of patients with hypertension often allows other medications to be discontinued earlier than otherwise.[9, 10] Its usefulness in treating heart attack victims was explored in a 1994 German study. Sixty-one patients with acute myocardial infarction were randomly assigned to two groups. One was treated with standard cardiac and blood pressure medications. The other group was treated with standard medications plus 100 mcg selenium and 100 mg CoQ10 per day. The patients were followed for one year. During that time 20 percent of the control group died from another heart attack but none of the treatment group did.[11]

A few weeks to several months are needed to see an effect, depending on dosage, which is usually in the 100 to 300 mg per day range, divided into two doses. The intestinal absorption of most preparations of CoQ10 is relatively poor—about 10 to 20 percent. This can be greatly enhanced by chewing the CoQ10 tablets or capsules with a spoonful of peanut butter or other fatty food.[12] The most dependable approach to adjusting dosage is to determine CoQ10 serum levels, which should be above 2 to 2.5 mcg per ml.[13] Although the availability of accurate CoQ10 lab tests currently is rather poor, this should improve over the next few years as CoQ10 therapy becomes more widespread.

Breast cancer may be molecularly caused by a dominant deficiency of vitamin Q10.[14] Researchers are working on treating breast cancer patients with CoQ10.[15]

Evidently, healthy people can benefit from CoQ10 as well. A 1997 double-blind study on Finnish skiers showed significant improvement in physical performance and recovery time with CoQ_{10} supplementation of 90 mg per day.[16]

Food Sources of CoQ_{10}

Organ meats (heart, liver, kidney), sardines, mackerel, beef, peanuts, and soy oil are among the best sources of dietary CoQ_{10}.[17]

Recommendations

No recommendation has been made.[18]

Woman's Guide Suggestion

Supplement with 30 to 50 mg daily.

Antagonists

CoQ_{10} is very sensitive to heat and light.

Toxicity

The toxicity levels are unknown.

10

Boron

PRIMARY FUNCTIONS

Promotes healthy bones
Increases absorption of calcium, magnesium, and phosphorus

BORON PLAYS A possible role in bone formation, and low boron consumption may be one of the factors involved in the development of osteoporosis. Boron is thought to be involved in parathyroid metabolism and thus influences the metabolism of calcium, magnesium, vitamin D,[1] and phosphorus.[2] Supplementation daily with 3 mg of boron markedly reduces the urinary loss of calcium and magnesium in postmenopausal women with boron-deficient diets. These changes are consistent with conservation of bone mass and resistance to osteoporosis. Interestingly, the supplementation also increased serum estradiol and testosterone levels. A well-balanced diet high in fruits and vegetables should be able to supply 1.5 to 3 mg of boron per day.[3]

Food Sources of Boron

Sources include green, leafy vegetables, grains, grapes, raisins, apples, nuts, wine, cider, and beer.

Recommendations

No RDA has been designated.

Woman's Guide Suggestion

Supplement with 3 mg of boron daily.

Toxicity

Environmental poisoning involving boric acid and borates has been reported.

11

Calcium

Primary Functions

Builds bones and teeth
Needed for proper heart rhythms
Needed to conduct nerve impulses
Needed for relaxation and contraction of muscle
May reduce risk of colon cancer
May lower blood pressure

Calcium is needed for the growth and health of bones and teeth. In fact, 99 percent of the body's calcium is stored in those tissues. Calcium stores reach maximum levels in the body somewhere between puberty and age 30. (See Chapter 23.) The stores are similar to a reservoir, the body filling the calcium reservoir for the first part of life and draining it in the second half. If there has been good nutrition and an adequate supply of calcium, the calcium reservoir should be large enough to last throughout life. Unfortunately, at the present time, no proven way has been found of catching up later in life if the reservoir runs low. It is critical, therefore, in the younger years, to consume a healthy diet high in calcium[1] and to maintain a moderate level of exercise to ensure good bone density.

Babies, young children, and adolescents need a lot of calcium; the major growth of our bones takes place in the early years. These bones must last us a lifetime. Until about age 60, the body absorbs about 30 percent of the dietary calcium consumed. After that the absorption declines. During pregnancy women use an additional 400 mg of calcium a day and when lactating an additional 300 mg per day.[2] The bad news is that the daily calcium intake for the average woman in the United States is generally less than half of the RDA of 800 mg.[3,4]

A few studies tried to determine if there are significant differences between the bone densities of vegetarian and omnivorous women. Results varied. In some studies, no significant differences between the groups were found.[5,6,7] Other studies found that vegetarians had greater bone density both before and after menopause.[8,9] One researcher found that vegetarian women lost 18 percent bone mass whereas the meat-eating women lost 35 percent after age 60.[10] It is known that red meat inhibits the absorption of calcium.

Many studies have been conducted to discover which minerals and vitamins are associated with high bone density. Zinc, iron, and magnesium appear to be indicators of high bone density in specific bone sites.[11] A study from North Dakota found that people in high fluoride areas had a lower incidence of osteoporosis and higher bone mineral density than in low fluoride areas.[12] This finding was supported by another study that compared two Finnish towns: Women in the town having fluoridated water had fewer bone fractures than women in the town without fluoridation.[13] In yet another study, groups of people who had been supplemented with a fluoride/calcium/vitamin D combination had the least number of fractures when they were compared with control groups.[14] Women with osteoporosis have been shown to be well below the RDAs in sodium, calcium, cholesterol, magnesium, fluoride, zinc, and folic acid. They also tend to have a very low caloric intake.[15]

As might be expected, women who have or have had *anorexia nervosa* (an eating disorder usually involving girls and women) have a significantly lower bone density than do women who eat normally. The low intake of nutrients along with the other typical behavior of the eating disorder cause accelerated bone loss.[16] Women on low-calorie diets may have decreased bone mineral density. (See Chapter 34.) It has been suggested that it is the quality of the total diet rather than solely the amount of calcium that prevents bone loss.[17]

Researchers reviewed 17 human trials that supported the hypothesis that calcium may exert chemoprotective effects. Calcium directly affects the cell cycle and increases the rates of cell differentiation, which may lower the risk of colon cancer.[18] In a large nurses' study, it was shown that a low intake of calcium is associated with an increased risk of colon cancer.[19] In a case-controlled study in Taiwan from 1989 through 1993, the causes of death were studied. The researchers indicated that calcium from drinking water had a protective effect against colon cancer.[20] Another study suggested the use of vitamin and mineral supplements, including calcium and vitamin E, was associated with reduced risk of colon cancer. Women who used multivitamins for 10 years had one-half the risk of colon cancer as individuals who did not use multivitamins.[21] In yet another study calcium and vitamin D were shown to lower the risk for colon cancer.[22] The 19-year study, which examined 1,954 men, found that the highest risk of colorectal cancer was seen in the group of men that had the lowest intakes of both vitamin D and calcium. The risk was reduced in each of the other three groups with higher intakes of the nutrients.[23]

Calcium, along with vitamin D, also appears to lower blood pressure. One study that examined 222 women aged 55 to 80 and 86 women aged 20 to 35 found that women who had less than the RDA in both calcium and vitamin D had significantly higher systolic blood pressure than women who met the RDA in one of the nutrients.[24]

Presently many women supplement their diets with calcium. The results of some studies indicate that if a person has a calcium deficiency and takes a calcium supplement, the bone mineral density is improved slightly. However, in those who do not have a calcium deficiency, calcium supplementation may not prevent bone loss due to menopause and aging.[25,26] Supporting calcium supplementation is a study that compared postmenopausal women over a two-year period. It found that women who were supplemented with 1,000 mg of calcium per day did have less bone loss than women who did not take a calcium supplement.[27]

Supplementation may also be more beneficial for slowing bone loss when it is combined with an exercise program.[28] In a study combining calcium intake and physical activity, it was found that bone mass in postmenopausal women was protected 5 to 12 years after menopause in all sites, including the spine and hip. High calcium consisted of more than 700 milligrams of calcium per day and physical activity consisted of at least 50 hours of physical activity per week.[29]

Based on the present information, chelated calcium and refined calcium carbonate tablets, calcium gluconate, calcium phosphate, and calcium citrate including antacids without aluminum may be safely and effectively ingested by most people. Individuals who have a family history of renal calcium stones may be concerned about calcium supplementation. Kidney stones affect 10 to 20 percent of adult Americans.[30] Most calcium supplements require an acidic environment in order to dissolve and be absorbed by the body. As people age, they generally produce less gastric acid, which is responsible for diminished calcium absorption. Different foods and juices can help to raise the acid levels. It may be a good idea to consume one of the acidic foods when taking a calcium supplement. Calcium carbonate requires an acidic environment to be dissolved and therefore should be taken with meals. Calcium phosphate is found in dairy products and some supplements. It is also dependent on an acidic environment for greater absorption. Calcium gluconate is absorbed by most people. However, it has less calcium per weight than some of the other calcium supplements. Calcium citrate requires less of an acidic environment for dissolution, which may lead to greater absorption.

Bonemeal and dolomite as nutritional supplements should be avoided. They may have other toxic ingredients such as lead and toxic metals.

Many people also use antacids as a calcium supplement. There are two problems in using an antacid. One, it is an antacid, and by definition it is designed to lessen gastric acidity, which can then reduce calcium absorption. Two, some antacids contain aluminum, which can leach the calcium out of the bones, causing it to be excreted.

Food Sources of Calcium

Sources include dairy products, soybean products, green, leafy vegetables, canned salmon with the bones, mackerel, sardines, raisins, and seaweed.

Recommendations

The RDA for calcium is 800 mg for women 25 and over. The RDA for pregnant and lactating women is 1,000 mg. Worldwide the recommended range varies from 400 to 1,000 mg per day.

Woman's Guide Suggestion

Under the age of 40 supplement with 1,000 to 1,500 mg of calcium daily, and over the age of 40 supplement with 1,500 to 2,000 mg daily.

Antagonists

Low levels of estrogen (after menopause) increase calcium loss. An alkaline stomach reduces the amount of calcium absorbed. Red meats, alcohol, and foods with oxalic acid impair the absorption of calcium. Sources of oxalic acid are beet greens, spinach, rhubarb, chard, and almonds. Anticoagulants, antiseizure medication, and extended use of cortisone put women at a higher risk of osteoporosis. High phosphorus intake may interfere with calcium absorption.

Toxicity

No adverse side effects have been reported with intakes of calcium as high as 2,500 mg per day. One exception is an increase in the incidence of urinary stones in males.[31]

Warning

Check with your doctor if you have kidney stones, kidney disease, or heart disease before supplementing with calcium. Calcium reduces the amount of iron absorption.[32]

12

Chromium

PRIMARY FUNCTIONS

Helps regulation of glucose metabolism
Aids synthesis of fatty acids and cholesterol
Used in protein transport
Lowers LDL and raises HDL blood levels
May protect against coronary artery disease

CHROMIUM HAS BEEN shown to be helpful in regulation of glucose metabolism, and deficiency has been determined to result in insulin resistance.[1] Individuals with some types of hypoglycemia have shown improvement in their laboratory indices as well as subjective symptoms, especially chilliness, after chromium supplementation.[2, 3] It is thought that these represent cases of chromium deficiency. Supplementation will generally not correct glucose metabolism diseases such as diabetes, but it may be helpful. Supplemental chromium was shown to have positive effects on glucose and insulin variables in individuals with Type 2 diabetes. Over the four-month period of the study, 200 mcg of chromium daily did not appear to be sufficient for the reversal of diabetic symptoms. However, 1,000 mcg of supplemental chromium daily had some affect.[4] Another study found that 500 mcg twice per day showed improvements.[5]

Trivalent chromium can lower the blood levels of low density lipoproteins (LDL, "bad cholesterol") and raise the high density lipoproteins (HDL, "good cholesterol").[6] Low levels of chromium also have been associated with higher risk of coronary heart disease.[7,8] Some suspicions have been raised recently that the association between alcohol consumption and reduced rates of heart disease may actually be due to the chromium content of yeast-fermented alcoholic beverages, not the alcohol content.

Chromium picolinate has become popular as a dietary supplement for weight reduction. Studies do not support this claim. (See Chapter 34.)

Chromium concentrations in body tissues decrease with age, and the parallel with age-related glucose intolerance may not be coincidental. Presently no readily available, accurate technique exists to determine chromium status in an individual, and therefore it is difficult to determine the necessary chromium requirement. Total body stores do not correlate with serum levels or with urine levels, and hair analysis is an unreliable indicator of chromium status in a given individual. Presently chromium deficiencies are best diagnosed in hindsight; that is, if a patient improves with supplementation, a retrospective diagnosis of chromium deficiency is made.

Chromium is a mineral found in the soil, and chromium-poor soil results in chromium-deficient foods. Processing foods and milling grains result in decreased amounts of chromium in the diet. Chromium losses are also increased by strenuous exercise, pregnancy, infection, and stress.[9,10]

Food Sources of Chromium

Brewer's yeast is high in chromium. However, care must be taken to be sure that the supplement is authentic brewer's yeast, as other sources such as baker's yeast do not contain significant amounts of chromium.[11] Other foods with chromium are wheat germ, whole grains, brown rice, beans, cheese, beer, and meat.

Recommendations

The RDA for a safe and adequate intake of chromium is between 50 and 200 mcg. Recently, chromium picolinate has been highly touted as a supplement, but some authorities doubt that it is superior to the less expensive chromium chloride or brewer's yeast. However, most diets contain less than 60 percent of the minimum suggested intake of 50 mcg.[12]

Woman's Guide Suggestion

Supplement with 80 mcg daily.

Antagonists

The processing of grains removes most of the chromium. Teflon-coated utensils and cookware other than stainless steel may reduce the amount of chromium in food.

Toxicity

Chromium has a large safety range, and no signs of toxicity have been found in the nutritional studies at levels up to 1 mg per day. In mining and industrial settings, industrial toxicity is caused by a different class of chromium compounds than are found in food or used for supplementation.

13

Copper

Primary Functions

Keeps blood vessels elastic
Needed for formation of elastin and collagen
Functions as an iron oxidizer
May increase risk of some cancers at high levels
Essential for proper functioning of vitamin C

Copper is an important iron-oxidizer, preventing free-radical formation. This helps prevent fats from becoming rancid or oxidizing.[1] This may be significant since it has been suggested that high iron blood levels may increase the risk of heart disease. (See Chapter 15.)

Elevated levels of copper have been found in patients with many different forms of cancer, including those of the female reproductive organs, bladder, large bowel, and stomach.[2] Other researchers suspect that there may be an increased risk of specific cancers associated with high copper and low zinc levels. In one study on 73 women hospitalized for suspected gynecological tumors, a correlation was found between the copper/zinc serum levels and tumor malignancies. The serum copper/zinc ratio was significantly higher in the malignant tumors than in the 48 benign growths. It was suggested that the copper/zinc ratio may be a marker for malignant tumors.[3] (See Chapter 22.)

The amount of copper we have in our daily diets is dependent on the amount of copper in the soil where the foods were grown and where the animals were grazed. Copper is absorbed by plants, ingested by animals, and ultimately consumed by people.

Food Sources of Copper

Sources include kidneys, shellfish, legumes, liver, nuts, bran, soybeans, and wheat germ.

Antagonists

Ascorbic acid inhibits copper absorption.[4] Copper works in conjunction with both zinc and vitamin C. High levels of either zinc or vitamin C will lower copper levels. Intravenous feeding commonly causes copper deficiencies.

Recommendations

The RDA subcommittee has stated a safe and adequate intake of copper is between 1.5 and 3 mg per day.[5]

Woman's Guide Suggestion

Supplement with 2 mg of copper daily.

Toxicity

Copper toxicity is rare in the United States. Most U.S. diets usually do not contain more than 5 mg per day with an occasional high of 10 mg per day.

Warning

People with Wilson's disease (a disorder of copper metabolism) should not take copper supplements without a physician's consultation.

14

Iodine

Primary Functions

Helps regulate metabolism of fats
Necessary for proper thyroid function
Reduces fibrocystic breast conditions

Iodine, which is turned into iodide in the body, has a significant role in the functioning of the thyroid gland. Iodine helps regulate metabolism, energy levels, and the burning of fat. There is evidence that increased iodine uptake increases the risk of the thyroid cancer papillary carcinoma, and iodine deficiencies may increase the risk of follicular carcinoma.[1]

Researchers in Canada and the United States have used different dosages and regimens of iodine to treat fibrocystic breast disease. They have found that all their patients were cyst-free and 70 percent were pain-free after four months of treatment. Within a year, 95 percent of the women found relief of pain. Long-standing fibrosis can take up to three years to eliminate.[2] Upon completion of testing four different types of iodine treatments on many women with fibrocystic disease, it was concluded that molecular iodine (I_2) was the most beneficial.[3]

Food Sources of Iodine

Sources include salt water fish, kelp, garlic, seasalt, mushrooms, soybeans, and summer squash.

Recommendations

The RDA for females ages 11 and up is 150 mcg. The RDA for pregnant women is 175 mcg; for lactating women it is 200 mcg.

Woman's Guide Suggestion

Supplement with 150 mcg of iodine daily.

Antagonists

Brussels sprouts, cabbage, pears, spinach, and turnips may inhibit iodine absorption if eaten in large quantities.

Toxicity

In Japan goiters have been induced by consuming large quantities of seaweed, which can contain 4.5 mg of iodine per gram dry weight. However, 1 to 2 mg of iodine per day have not resulted in any adverse physiological problems in healthy adults.[4]

15

Iron

Primary Function

Necessary for production of hemoglobin and myoglobin (hemoglobin's twin in muscle tissue)
May increase risk of heart disease at high levels
May increase risk of infections at high or low levels

Iron is a very controversial mineral. On one hand, it has been reported that up to 20 million Americans suffer from anemia,[1] much of it the result of iron deficiency. On the other hand, there is now great concern that high levels of iron may be partly responsible for heart and liver disease. Iron is stored in the body by specialized proteins called *ferritin* and used as it is needed. As the levels of stored iron increase so does extra, free-floating iron. When the free iron comes in contact with oxygen, it accelerates chemical reactions in the body, causing oxidation damage to cell walls.[2]

Iron requirements are higher for women who are menstruating, pregnant, or lactating and lower for women postmenopausally. Menstruating women have iron stores of about 200 to 300 mg. After menopause, the iron stores increase (as well as the risk of heart disease) to approximately 800 mg—similar to that of men. Dr. Lauffer, researcher and author of *Iron Balance*, suggests that it would be best to keep the iron stores between 100 and 400 mg.[3] Another group of researchers reviewed 7 epidemiology studies and found a positive association between coronary heart disease and ferritin levels. They also reviewed 18 epidemiology studies and found no association between coronary heart disease and ferritin levels. The iron hypothesis remains unproven.[4,5] One of the limitations in reviewing the iron literature is a lack of agreed-upon parameters for assessing the iron status in humans. More studies are needed to assess the iron/coronary heart disease association.[6]

Iron stores can be reduced by regularly giving blood. Also walking, although the exact length and amount necessary is unknown, has been shown to reduce serum ferritin levels in postmenopausal women.[7] Depending on your age, beware; there is a great deal of iron fortification in food in the United States and most multiple vitamins contain iron.

Researchers have attempted to tie both high and low levels of iron to increased rates of infection, but the studies are controversial, and laboratory abnormalities appear to be more impressive than clinical evidence in humans. An exception should probably be made for iron supplementation in endemic malaria areas, in which supplementation is followed by an increase in acute disease. [8,9]

Food Sources of Iron

Red meats, fortified cereals and breads, fish, green, leafy vegetables, poultry, and beans are good sources of iron. Additionally, alcohol and vitamin C enhance iron absorption.

Recommendations

The RDA for women between the ages of 25 and 50 is 15 mg and for women 50 and above 10 mg. The RDA for pregnant women is 30 mg; for lactating women it is 15 mg.

Woman's Guide Suggestion

Under the age of 40, supplement with 15 mg of iron daily, and over the age of 40, supplement with 9 mg daily.

Antagonists

Phytates, chemical compounds found in unprocessed grains, prevent absorption of iron.

Toxicity

Iron intake between 25 and 75 mg per day has not caused problems in healthy adults. Taking 200 to 250 mg per kg of body weight in one dose can be lethal. Approximately 2,000 cases of iron poisoning occur yearly in the United States. These reported cases are mostly in children who take their parents' adult iron supplements.

Warning

High levels of iron postmenopausally have been suggested to increase the risk of heart disease. Inorganic iron can inhibit vitamin E absorption. A small population of people with idiopathic hemochromatosis is genetically at risk for iron overload. They absorb iron very efficiently into the body and can suffer from chronic iron toxicity, leading to heart and liver damage.

16

Magnesium

Primary Functions

Involved in more than 330 enzymatic reactions[1]
Needed for bone formation and growth
May prevent bone loss
Act as coronary artery relaxant
May prevent heart disease
Aids in managing pre-eclampsia (a hypertensive disorder of pregnancy), treating cardiac arrhythmias,[2] and managing diabetes[3]
May lower blood pressure

Magnesium plays a significant role in the formation and structure of bones. The body contains about 25 gr of magnesium and 50 to 60 percent of that is in the bones.[4] People in the United States had a higher magnesium intake in their diets at the beginning of the century than they do presently. Today the American diet contains less grain than it did in the past, and the grain we do eat has had most of its magnesium removed by milling.[5] In America all age groups consume less than the RDA of magnesium.[6, 7]

It appears that magnesium metabolism changes postmenopausally and after an oophorectomy, or ovariectomy. When the estrogen levels drop, an increased excretion of magnesium occurs. Estrogen restores the magnesium levels by increasing intestinal absorption. In a study based on the NHANES I, investigators looked at the serum magnesium levels of 224 pregnant women, 1,559 nonpregnant women taking birth control pills, 2,884 postmenopausal women between the ages of 50 and 74, and 4,145 nonpregnant women in a control group between the ages of 15 and 49. The investigators found that pregnant women and women on the pill had reduced magnesium serum levels when compared to the control group. Postmenopausal women had the highest serum magnesium levels.[8]

Other researchers, examining the role of magnesium and bone loss, compared different ERT/HRT hormone treatments taken by postmenopausal women and compared the results to a control group. The results of the study indicated that the women who took estrogen with a progestogen decreased their urinary excretion of magnesium.[9] Although the exact role of magnesium and bone loss is not clear, the researchers indicated that low levels of magnesium may be one of the factors that contribute to osteoporosis. It was also stated that the present recommended magnesium intake may be too low.

A study that specifically looked at the relationship between magnesium and calcium found an interesting result. It followed postmenopausal women who were taking varied and different types of ERT/HRT. The women who took 500 mg of calcium and 1,000 mg of magnesium reversed their bone loss. A significant increase in bone mineral density occured within a year. Because the bulk of the research does not support calcium megadosing in the postmenopausal years, it was suggested that there should be a change in the RDA levels of both calcium and magnesium. The authors suggested raising the magnesium levels to 1,000 mg per day and lowering the calcium levels to 500 mg per day.[10] Further research is being conducted with women not taking ERT/HRT to see if they also have reduced bone loss with higher magnesium intakes.

Magnesium, vitamin D, phosphorus, sodium, potassium, manganese, and calcium all interact. The optimal ratios among these agents are not known, but it is assumed that a balance is critical for bone formation and health. It is generally accepted that about a 1 to 3 ratio of magnesium to calcium be maintained. However, as pointed out previously, some researchers are advocating the reverse of this ratio.

There has also been interest in magnesium's role in ischemic (coronary) heart disease. Magnesium is important as a coronary artery relaxant, and it is necessary for normal cardiac electrical function. Many different heart problems have been attributed to magnesium deficiencies. Low levels of magnesium are associated with abnormal heart rhythms and sudden death ischemic heart disease,[11, 12] and intravenous magnesium given to acute heart attack patients has shown reductions in death and morbidity.[13] Reviews of epidemiological and geographical studies show that areas with low magnesium levels in the water and the soil have higher death rates from ischemic heart disease.[14]

Studies have been done on the prevalence of heart disease in geographic areas having hard or soft water supplies. Hard water has more calcium and magnesium than does soft water. Water softeners replace the calcium and magnesium with sodium. (High sodium levels may be a problem for some people.) It has been found that individuals who drink soft water have lower levels of magnesium in their cardiac muscle. They also have a higher incidence of sudden death ischemic heart disease.[15]

It has been shown that magnesium supplementation may lower blood pressure and also improve serum lipids. High concentrations of HDL and low concentrations of LDL along with low blood pressure reduce mortality from strokes and ischemic heart disease. In a study of 33 people, 23 of those people received a magnesium supplement and 10 received a placebo. The men were given 548 milligrams of magnesium three times a day for four weeks, and the women were given 411 milligrams of magnesium for four weeks. The magnesium supplementation reduced blood pressure and improved lipid metabolism.[16]

Intracellular magnesium may play an important role in modulating insulin-mediated glucose uptake and vascular tone. People with non-insulin-dependent diabetes mellitus and who are hypertensive tend to have lower intracellular magnesium concentrations.[17]

Food Sources of Magnesium

Green vegetables, seafood, legumes, nuts, meats, and many dairy products provide magnesium. Most of the magnesium has been removed from processed grains.

Recommendation

The RDA for women over 25 is 280 mg. The RDA for pregnant women is 300 mg; for lactating women in the first six months it is 355 mg, and 340 mg from six months on. Magnesium gluconate is commonly used as a supplement.

Woman's Guide Suggestion

Under the age of 40, supplement with 400 to 600 mg of magnesium daily; after the age of 40, supplement with 500 to 700 mg daily.

Antagonists

High levels of calcium can interfere with magnesium absorption. Diabetes, heart problems, alcoholism, cirrhosis, any trauma to the body, and any malabsorption problems can interfere with magnesium absorption.[18] Diuretics can inhibit magnesium absorption.

Toxicity

Presently no evidence exists that high levels of magnesium causes any serious problems except as noted below in cases of heart or kidney disease.

Warning

Large doses of magnesium will work as a laxative. People who have kidney problems or cardiac patients who have heart block should talk with their physicians before using a magnesium supplement.

17

Manganese

Primary Functions

Needed for bone growth
May help prevent osteoporosis
Regulates production and release of insulin
Metabolizes fats and proteins
Necessary for nerve transmission
Used in production of mother's milk
Aids in production of thyroxin (thyroid gland hormone)

MANGANESE IS necessary for bone growth and may play a part in preventing osteoporosis. Recent studies on osteoporosis showed that women with the disease had manganese levels from 29 to 75 percent below that of controls.[1,2] Manganese absorption is a problem in that many high-manganese foods also contain agents that inhibit manganese absorption. Calcium supplementation (as for osteoporosis prevention) can also decrease manganese absorption from the diet.

Food Sources of Manganese

Sources include whole grains, nuts, vegetables, fruits, milk, meats, and eggs.

Recommendations

The RDA's provisional level is set between 2 and 5 mg per day.

Woman's Guide Suggestion

Supplement with 5 mg of manganese daily.

Antagonists

Large amounts of calcium, phosphorus, magnesium, and phytates (found in whole grains), tannins, and oxalic acids will inhibit absorption.

Toxicity

The only toxicity reported has been from environmental exposure rather than dietary.

Warning

Women with low manganese levels may be at risk for increased iron loss due to menstrual bleeding.[3]

18

Molybdenum

PRIMARY FUNCTIONS

Metabolizes fats
Plays a biochemical role in functioning of enzymes
Plays a role in iron utilization

MANY RESEARCHERS state that molybdenum supplementation is unnecessary unless food comes from soil deficient in the mineral. Individuals who have a deficiency in molybdenum may have an increased incidence of esophageal cancer.[1]

Food Sources of Molybdenum

Milk, beans, breads, whole grains, legumes, and organ meat provide molybdenum.

Recommendations

The RDA for a safe and adequate intake of molybdenum is 75 to 250 mcg. The daily requirements of this element can be met in the daily diet. The public water supply usually provides 2 to 8 mcg daily.

Woman's Guide Suggestion

Supplement with 15 mcg of molybdenum daily.

Antagonists

Sulfate may inhibit the absorption of molybdenum. Molybdenum and copper in the intestinal tract form a compound that inhibits the absorption of both elements. This is modified by dietary sulfur.

Toxicity

Ten mg per day of molybdenum has produced toxic reactions; 0.54 mg per day has resulted in copper loss in the urine.

19

Phosphorus

Primary Functions

Needed for formation of bones and teeth
Necessary for muscle contraction
Assists kidney functions
Necessary for nervous system transmission

Phosphorus is a part of every cell in the body, but it is especially necessary for the formation of bones and teeth. Approximately 85 percent of phosphorus is found in the bones. A balance between phosphorus and calcium intakes is important. A ratio of dietary calcium to phosphorus less than 1 to 2 may cause a lowered calcium blood level. In some animal studies a low calcium-to-phosphorus ratio leads to bone resorption.[1] People who consume little in the way of dairy products and green vegetables can have a calcium-to-phosphorus ratio as low as 1 to 4.

Foods Rich in Phosphorus

Phosphorus is contained in almost all foods but is very high in both sodas and red meats. Most "junk foods" are high in phosphorus and should be avoided.

Recommendations

The RDA for women age 25 and above is 800 mg; for pregnant and lactating women it is 1,200 mg.

Woman's Guide Suggestion

Supplementation is not necessary since adequate amounts of phosphorus are consumed in the diet.

Antagonists

Aluminum hydroxide, found in some antacids, inhibits absorption.

Toxicity

There is no known toxic level. However, high levels of phosphorus in animals causing calcium-to-phosphorus ratios less than 1 to 2 have resulted in bone resorption.

Warning

Phosphorus levels in normal diets in the United States are not thought to be dangerous to humans, especially if there is adequate intake of calcium and vitamin D.[2]

20

Potassium

Primary Functions

Reduces risk of strokes
Maintains good blood pressure
Needed for transmission of nerve impulses
Needed for proper muscle contraction

A ubiquitous element in virtually all living cells, potassium is a key constituent of the "internal ocean" of salts in which our tissues live. It is necessary in one way or another for almost any function of any tissue, but especially for nerve transmission and muscle contraction.

A 1987 study, done over a 12-year period, found that men and women who consumed a high potassium diet suffered fewer strokes. One extra serving of a fresh vegetable or fruit per day was associated with a 40 percent reduced risk of stroke-associated mortality.[1]

Recommendations

The National Research Council states that the minimum potassium requirement is between 1,600 and 2,000 mg per day. However, ingesting 3,500 mg per day may have a beneficial effect on hypertension (high blood pressure). The council recommends an additional intake of fruits and vegetables. There was no recommendation for increased levels for pregnant or lactating women.[2]

Woman's Guide Suggestion

Supplementation of potassium is not necessary since adequate amounts are consumed in the diet.

Food Sources of Potassium

Fruits, vegetables, fresh meats, legumes, fish, and whole grains provide potassium.

Antagonists

Processed foods often have decreased potassium and increased sodium. Alcohol and coffee cause potassium loss.

Toxicity

Eighteen grams of potassium a day can cause acute intoxication and death by cardiac arrest. Lesser amounts normally harmless to someone with normal kidneys may result quickly in fatal hyperkalemia (high potassium blood levels) in persons with chronic kidney failure.

Warning

Some diuretics and extended periods of vomiting or diarrhea will deplete potassium. As noted in Toxicity, increased intake of potassium is dangerous to persons with renal failure.

21

Selenium

Primary Functions

Acts as antioxidant
Reduces risk of heart attack and heart disease
Reduces risk of cancers
Protects against metal poisoning
Synergistic with vitamin E

Selenium is a trace mineral in the soil. Fruits, vegetables, and grains have varying selenium contents depending on the selenium levels in the soil in which they grew. It has been reported that the most selenium-poor soil in the United States is around the Great Lakes, most of the east coast, and the west coast. These areas are also reported to have the highest incidence of breast cancer.[1]

Research studies have shown a relationship between low selenium levels and an increased risk of myocardial infarction. One study, which examined 84 patients with heart problems and 84 without, found significantly lower serum selenium levels in patients with myocardial infarction. The patients had low levels of selenium in their toenails, which indicated that the low selenium levels preceded the heart attacks.[2, 3] Today, after 20 years of research, the results of the longitudinal studies concerning selenium and cardiovascular disease are still conflicting. Some studies have found a relationship between low selenium levels and a higher risk of coronary disease. However, others have not found an association.[4] In a 1994 randomized, controlled trial using selenium, 100 mcg per day with CoQ10 demonstrated a significant reduction in heart attack deaths in the treatment group.[5] (See Chapter 9.)

A comparison of people with high and low selenium blood levels in China encountered many fewer cases of esophageal, stomach, and liver cancers among subjects with higher levels of selenium.[6]

A Finnish four-year prospective study ending in 1980 determined that low selenium and low vitamin E levels were significantly associated with increased cancer death rates in men.[7]

Another study compared two groups of 30 healthy postmenopausal women from both Finland and Japan. Finland has a high incidence of coronary heart disease, breast cancer, and endometrial (uterine lining) cancer compared to Japan. Finland is also a selenium-poor country compared to Japan. The researchers compared selenium, vitamin A, vitamin E, and cholesterol levels. The findings showed no differences in serum vitamin A levels, but the Finns had higher vitamin E and cholesterol and lower serum selenium levels than did the Japanese.[8] It was suggested that these vitamin and selenium variations could account for the differences in risk of heart disease and cancer between the two countries.

The exact relationship between selenium and vitamin E is unknown, but the two are interdependent. One of the above groups found a synergistic relationship between low selenium and vitamin E levels as a predictive marker for cancer death.[9] In addition, a few deficiency diseases can be reversed by therapy with either selenium or vitamin E.[10]

Selenium has also been shown to protect the body against silver, mercury, and cadmium toxicity.[11]

Food Sources of Selenium

Seafood, liver, kidneys, grains, chicken, egg yolk, mushrooms, and garlic provide selenium.

Recommendations

The RDA for women over 25 is 55 mcg. The RDA for pregnant women is 65 mcg; for lactating women it is 75 mcg.

Woman's Guide Suggestion

Supplement with of 50 mcg of selenium daily.

Toxicity

Chronic intake of 5 mg has caused hair loss and fingernail changes.[12]

22

Zinc

Primary Functions

Required trace element of DNA and RNA
Needed for growth and sexual development
Required for proper alcohol metabolism

Zinc is needed by virtually all plants and animals. It is a critical component for children's growth and sexual development. Important during pregnancy and lactation, zinc is a necessary nutrient for fetal development. Zinc deficiency has been associated with abnormalities in taste, poor wound healing, skin lesions, and immune dysfunction.[1]

Assessing zinc status in people is difficult. Zinc deficiency is often covert until it results in an obvious problem. Researchers have shown that postmenopausal women showed no significant change in serum zinc levels even after four months of relative zinc deprivation. This is despite the fact that more sophisticated assays of zinc-dependent function indicated a decrease in activity that was corrected by zinc supplementation. The conclusion was that zinc levels in the blood may not be a reliable indicator of deficiency states. An overt problem due to zinc deficiency may appear before detection is possible, especially in the elderly, who are more prone to zinc deficiencies than younger people.[2] However, data from the Nationwide Food Consumption Survey, Continuing Survey of Food Intakes found that zinc intakes of teenage girls, adult women, young children, and elderly often fall short of the RDA.[3]

Alcoholics generally have low levels of zinc. This may be due to an inadequate diet or due to alcohol inhibiting zinc absorption. This may be a compounded problem since low zinc levels decrease the body's ability to metabolize alcohol, resulting in prolonged exposure to high alcohol levels and increased tissue damage.[4,5]

Estrogen in pre- and postmenopausal women lowers zinc levels in the blood. It also raises the copper to levels similar to those seen in pregnant women. Some researchers have concluded that a progestogen should be added to postmenopausal hormone treatments to balance the copper to zinc ratios.[6]

Food Sources of Zinc

Oysters, meats, poultry, and some vegetables provide zinc. Breast milk and zinfandel wine enhance the bioavailability of zinc.

Recommendations

The RDA for women 25 and above is 12 mg. The RDA for pregnant women is 15 mg; for lactating women in the first six months it is 19 mg and then drops to 16 mg.

Woman's Guide Suggestion

Under the age of 40, supplement with 20 mg of zinc daily. After 40, supplement with 30 mg daily.

Antagonists

Phytates, high fiber diets, tin, oxalate, copper, and possibly high phosphorus intake inhibit zinc absorption. Vegetarians, athletes, and dieters tend to have lower levels of zinc. It appears that the bioavailability of zinc is dependent on the total diet, and all of its antagonists are not clearly understood.

Toxicity

Zinc in the amount of 18.5 mg per day has been shown to create an impairment of copper metabolism. Large doses of 2 g or more can acutely cause nausea and vomiting. Immune function has been depressed by 300 mg per day of zinc.[7] Chronically taking more than 10 times the RDA can result in many problems.[8]

Part III

Topics of Prime Concern to Women

23

Bones

BONES ARE MADE up of 70 percent mineral and 30 percent organic components. The organic matter is mostly collagen, and the minerals are largely calcium and phosphorus salts. There are two types of bone tissue: cortical and trabecular. *Cortical* bone tissue forms the outer shell of the bone and is mostly found in the shafts of long bones such as the humerus (arm) and femur (thigh). *Trabecular* bone is the porous bone tissue mostly found in the vertebrae (backbone), the flat bones (face, pelvis, skull), and the distal (far) ends of the long bones. However, in many locations throughout the body, bones contain both cortical and trabecular bone in varying proportion.

Bones go through a regular growth pattern consisting of stages of bone resorption and bone remodeling, called *bone turnover*. The first stage of resorption begins with *osteoclasts* (specialized bone demolition cells) dissolving some of the bone tissue and leaving an excavated or dug-out area in the bone. In the next stage, the *osteoblasts* (bone construction cells) begin rebuilding a collagen framework for new bone in the excavated areas. The osteoblasts continue rebuilding until there is mineralization of the bone and then go into a resting stage. Up to 10 percent of the bone throughout the body is actively involved in these different stages at the same time. The entire resorption and remodeling process takes about 100 days to complete. Under the best of conditions in adulthood, the bone remodeling and bone resorption are equal to one another and no net bone loss occurs until menopause.

In a normal, healthy person until the approximate age of 35 to 40, the cortical bones keep developing to reach peak mass. It has been thought that trabecular bones reach their peak mass at about the age of 25 to 30 years.[1] However, some of the newer studies suggest that 86 percent of peak bone mass is achieved before menarche and in the two years following (i.e., before age 14). For all practical purposes, adult bone density seems to be reached by age 17 in females.[2, 3] Regardless, sometime in early adulthood the bones stop building and begin to decline. Generally, a woman does not have any significant bone loss until menopause unless she has specific health problems, develops amenorrhea (stops menstruating) due to excessive exercise, has anorexia nervosa, or does not eat properly. Any of these conditions can lead to an increased risk of osteoporosis.

Bone loss becomes problematic at menopause. Hormonal changes accelerate bone loss for approximately one decade. At that point the bone loss returns to a slower, age-related loss rate similar to that of men. At about the age of 40, a woman will lose approximately 0.3 to 0.4 percent of her total bone mass each year. After menopause the bone loss may accelerate up to 2 to 3 percent of the entire bone mass each year.[4]

ERT/HRT still offers one the best methods of preventing bone loss in postmenopausal women. The treatment should begin at menopause and be continued for a minimum of 7 to 10 years, or indefinitely, in order to reduce long-term fracture rates.[5, 6] As soon as the treatment stops, the bone density drops. Also, many side effects of ERT/HRT exist. (See Chapter 25.) New drugs are being developed all the time. Recent studies indicate that natural progesterone creams, along with a good diet, nutrients, and exercise, appear to stop bone loss and actually increase bone density.[7]

Osteoporosis

Osteoporosis is a disease characterized by a reduction of bone mass that leads to a bone fracture(s). Both cortical and trabecular bones become weakened and are unable to withstand stresses of normal, daily life. Microscopically, the bones take on the appearance of Swiss cheese. Some women develop a dowager's hump. The spinal vertebrae become so porous that their collapse creates the characteristic pronounced hump on the upper back.

Worldwide, osteoporosis is more of a problem in urban, highly industrialized areas.[8] It is less prevalent in locations where diets contain whole grains, fish, tofu, and seaweed. Except for women who are on estrogen supplementation, all postmenopausal women experience higher rates of bone loss than other healthy people; it is not known why some women develop actual osteoporosis and some do not. Hormone supplementation reduces the amount of calcium lost and delays the menopausal bone loss.[9, 10, 11] But it should be noted that this therapy is not without risk. (See Chapter 25.)

Osteoporosis affects approximately 25 million people, mostly women, in the United States each year. The disease results in approximately 1.5 million fractures each year.[12] One-third of all women will have fractures by the time they are 65, and one-third of women by extreme old age will have a fractured hip.[13] Although fewer than 2 percent of women over the age of 65 will die from osteoporosis-related hip fractures,[14] the morbidity, pain, and related expense of fractures are staggering. The mortality rate for people in the first year after a hip fracture is 12 to 20 percent higher than for people without fractures.[15] The total cost for caring for people with osteoporosis, both directly and indirectly, is estimated at $18 billion a year.[16]

Osteoporosis has been categorized as either primary (type I) or secondary (type II). Type I osteoporosis affects women after menopause. It mainly affects the trabecular bone, which leads to many spinal fractures. An estimated 5 to 10 percent of women get osteoporosis[17] marked by a spinal fracture within the first 15 to 20 years after menopause. Type II osteoporosis generally affects women over 70 years old. It is an age-related bone loss and affects both the cortical and the trabecular bones.[18]

Postmenopausal women are also at the highest risk for requiring major dental work. Osteoporosis plays a large role in deterioration of the teeth and jaw bone structure, which makes dental work difficult.[19, 20] One source stated that by age 60 approximately 40 percent of women will have lost their teeth. The author had not resolved the question of whether the loss of teeth was due to poor dental care, osteoporosis, or a combination of the two.[21]

Exercise

Exercise has been shown to play a large role both in bone growth and in retarding bone loss. Weight-bearing exercise, aerobic dance, walking, and exercise that involves full-range motions have been shown to be the most beneficial.[22, 23] It appears that 20 to 45 minutes of moderate exercise such as dancing, aerobics, and jogging is effective in helping to maintain bone density.[24, 25] A new study of more than 200 women indicates that walking over a mile daily as regular exercise is associated with a greater overall bone density. However, although walking appeared to reduce the rate of bone loss from the legs, it had no effect on bone loss from other areas of the skeleton.[26] A different group concluded after a two-year follow-up of 65 postmenopausal women not on estrogen or hormone replacement therapy that non-weight-bearing exercises were ineffective in reducing vertebral bone loss.[27] However, falls and the fractures they cause are major causes of death in elderly women in the United States. Any exercise that increases muscle tone, balance, and agility will also help to reduce the risk in falling.[28]

Physical activity is important in maximizing a woman's genetic potential for good bone mineral density. Even a small gain of bone mineral density may have a considerable effect on preventing osteoporosis and reducing fractures.[29] In a study of bone health in mother-daughter pairs, the hormonal factors and behavior factors appeared to have a greater effect on bone mineral density than did familial associations. The good news is that women may successfully enhance their genetically determined bone mass by weight-bearing exercise, postmenopausal ERT, and adequate calcium intake.[30]

Exercise also is known to help cardiovascular health, gastrointestinal health, and psychological health. Yet, the benefits gained from exercise are short-lived and reversible.[31] When physical activity and stress on bone and muscles are eliminated, the bone mineral density decreases.[32] It has been shown that people who are immobile or bedridden have a large loss of bone in a short time. Exercise needs to be a part of a lifelong routine.

Mineral and Vitamin Intake

Calcium intake and exercise together were shown to protect overall bone mass in postmenopausal women 5 to 12 years after menopause. Dietary calcium intake of more than 700 mg per day and regular exercise of at least 50 hours physical activity per week has been shown to protect overall bone mass in postmenopause.[33]

Studies on the value of calcium supplementation after menopause are conflicting.[34, 35, 36, 37] Some studies say calcium supplementation has no effect on risk of fractures, and others say it is effective. However, in general, the majority of researchers recommend that young women consume a diet high in calcium, that premenopausal women supplement their diets with 1,000 to 1,500 mg of calcium per day, that postmenopausal women not on estrogen or hormone replacement therapy supplement their diets with 1,500 to 2,000 mg of calcium per day, and that postmenopausal women on estrogen or hormone replacement therapy supplement their diets with 1,000 to 1,500 mg of calcium per day. Based on the present information, chelated calcium and refined calcium carbonate tablets, including antacids, may be safely ingested by most people at doses not to exceed 2,000 milligrams per day. Calcium is also better absorbed in the evening before bed.[38] Individuals who have a family history of renal calcium stones may be concerned about calcium supplementation. Kidney stones affect 10 to 20 percent of adult Americans.[39]

Other research shows that calcium, 1,000 to 1,500 mg, along with vitamin D, at least 400 IU, per day intake is the key to maintaining bone health,[40] that one without the other doesn't work. In two large studies, supplementation of calcium and vitamin D decreased fractures over a four-year period by 30 to 70 percent.[41] Another study of women and men, over 65, who were given 500 mg of calcium and 700 IU of vitamin D3 showed decreased bone loss in the femoral neck, spine, and total body over a three-year period. The treatment reduced the incidence of non-vertebral fractures.[42] However, some question exists concerning the long-term effects of taking vitamin D. It appears to have some negative effects on lipid profiles.[43]

In one study, postmenopausal women given ipriflavone at 600 mg per day prevented the increase in bone turnover and decreased bone density that follows ovarian failure. These were the same results as in women given ipriflavone at 400 milligrams and conjugated estrogens at .3 mg a day.[44] The question still remains: What is the optimal combination for each person?

Obviously, other minerals and vitamins play an enormous role in achieving peak bone density. Researchers are looking at individual agents as well combinations that either enhance or decrease bone health. Dietary protein intake may be a determining factor in achieving peak bone mass in premenopausal but not in postmenopausal white women. Low intakes of protein, calcium, and phosphorus resulted in young women having more fractures. Also, diets high in meat protein promote excretion of calcium. However, researchers suggested that women who consume high protein diets may also consume diets high in calcium.[45] According to the 1989–1991 Continuing Surveys of Food Intakes by Individuals, conducted by the U.S. Department of Agriculture, phosphorus intake in the United States is high relative to calcium. Calcium intakes do not meet the 1989 RDAs for the age group of 10 and over, whereas phosphorus intake exceeds the RDA for most age groups. Eating processed food, especially junk food, increases phosphorus intake. High phosphorus intake may possibly interfere with vitamin D and calcium homoeostasis.[46] Other researchers compared current and past dietary intakes and bone mineral densities of 994 healthy premenopausal women between 45 and 49 years of age. They found that long-term intakes of vitamin C, zinc, magnesium, potassium, and fiber result in higher bone mineral density. A diet rich in fruits and vegetables appears to improve bone health. A possible connection to acid-base balance exists.[47] The American Academy of Rheumatology now recommends 800 IU of vitamin D daily for postmenopausal women.

Maintaining Bone Health

Major factors in maintaining bone health for premenopausal women are listed in order of decreasing importance: active ovarian function, physical activity, calcium intake, body size, low alcohol consumption, and a lack of cigarette smoking. In postmenopausal women, the factors that proved most important are calcium intake and physical activity.[48]

Many factors put a women at higher risk of osteoporosis:

- Fair complexion
- Old age
- Early menopause or surgical menopause (reduction of estrogen)
- Amenorrhea (reduction of estrogen)
- A thin body build (below 15 percent body fat is high risk) and lean body mass[49]
- Caucasian or Asian race
- Positive family history
- Drugs (e.g., corticosteroids, thyroxine)
- Low calcium diet
- Smoking cigarettes
- High alcohol consumption
- Physical inactivity
- Specific health problems
- Low nutrient absorption in postmenopausal women[50]
- Prematured hair graying, which has been associated with low bone density.[51]
- Past or current depression in women (Bone mineral density in depressed women was on average 6 to 14 percent less than women who were not depressed.[52])

In summary, for good bone health:

- Achieve as much bone mass as possible before age 15.
- Eat a well-balanced diet high in calcium.
- Supplement with calcium, vitamin D, magnesium, boron, manganese, and phosphorus.
- Take regular exercise, both aerobic and weight-bearing.
- Possibly take ERT/HRT.[53]
- Be aware of medications that reduce bone density, such as steroids, anticoagulants, and anticonvulsants.
- Eat foods high in acids (e.g., citrus, tomatoes, cranberry juice, vinegars), which improve calcium absorption.
- Avoid carbonated soda beverages, as these contain high levels of phosphate and interfere with calcium absorption.

- Eat green vegetables. They are good sources of calcium, 52 to 60 percent of which is absorbed.
- Increase tea consumption, which has been associated with high bone mineral density in hip and spine.[54]

Screening

Bone mineral density can be measured by different methods. Four commonly used methods are: tomography, single photon and dual-photon absorptiometry, and the newer technique of dual-energy X-ray absorbtiometry. The tests use a small amount of radiation exposure, less than 5 millirem (mrem) per study, and are accurate to within 1 or 2 percent. Bone measurements can be used to establish a baseline, determine risk, prescribe treatment, and evaluate treatment effectiveness. The bone measurement costs approximately $200. Specific bone density studies are necessary because, unfortunately, 30 to 40 percent of bone mass must be lost before osteoporosis is apparent on most X-rays.

Bone sonometry, using quantitive ultrasound, can also help in the diagnosis and assessment of osteoporosis. It measures the speed of sound propagation in bone, which in turn provide a measurement of bone density and strength. It is a non-invasive procedure that does not use radiation and costs approximately $40. Some sonometers have excellent accuracy and reproducibility, and others do not.

A single assessment by one of the above methods gives a snapshot of bone density at a single point in time, but it does not show whether bone is currently being lost or gained, or whether it is stable. Only serial studies over months and years will show a trend. However, urine tests are now available[55] for assessing current bone metabolism. They measure the collagen cross-links, deoxypridinoline, and N-telopeptide (Ntx), which are indicators of bone resorption.

After menopause, a bone density study should be done on women with a family history of osteoporosis or a history of disease or medication associated with rapid bone loss, and the study should be repeated at three- to five-year intervals.[56] Also, healthy postmenopausal women who are fast bone losers can be identified by measuring the lumbar bone mineral density along with a few biochemical determinations. This should be repeated twice in a six-month interval. It is a great preventive measure for identifying women at high risk for developing osteoporosis and fractures.[57]

Treatment

Osteoporosis therapy is evolving rapidly. A few years ago, no treatment was available. Now, along with calcium supplementation, we have estrogen (the most commonly used agent), calcitonin, and the bisphosphonates. Calcitonin (Miacalcin[58]), available in the United States as an injection or nasal spray, represented a major advance in therapy.[59] It increases bone strength and diminishes the pain of vertebral compression fractures. It was the only FDA approved treatment for osteoporosis until the approval of the bisphosphonate drug alendronate (Fosamax[60]). Fosamax has been shown to not only increase bone mass but prevent fractures. It is now considered the premiere agent for the treatment of osteoporosis. Other bisphosphonates include etidronate (Didronel[61]), pamidronate (Aredia[62]), and residronate (Actonel[63]). Didronel was originally used to treat hypercalcemia (high calcium blood levels) associated with malignancies. It also increases bone density and is thus helpful with osteoporosis, but it has been largely supplanted by newer drugs like Fosamax. Aredia is often used in cases where the patient is intolerant to Fosamax and where Miacalcin is not adequate to treat the severity of the osteoporosis. Residronate is approved for treatment of Paget's disease of the bone, but not yet approved for osteoporosis. In addition to these, insulin-like growth factors look like hopeful future therapies. These growth factors improve bone density by increasing osteoblastic (bone building) activity. Bisphosphonates and estrogen work by impeding osteoclastic (bone resorption) activity. The selective estrogen receptor modulators (SERMS) show promise for the future as well.

The treatment of osteoporosis is not an either/or therapy. Frequently, especially in severe cases, combination therapy consisting of estrogen, a bisphosphonate such as Fosamax, and Miacalcin may be used together.

An effective osteoporosis treatment must increase bone density, decrease fracture rate, and improve quality of life. More agents fitting this description will be available in the next few decades. Even today osteoporosis is preventable, and it is treatable even in severe cases.

24

Cancer

CANCER IS A number of different diseases grouped together by their characteristic behavior: Abnormal cells grow in an uncontrolled manner and spread. Cancer is caused by diverse influences, including intrinsic and extrinsic factors. Many of these factors are unknown, but among the known factors are various chemicals, radiation, viruses, hormones, immune dysfunctions, and individual genetic predispositions.

Cancers from six sites represent the majority of cancer cases and cause half the deaths due to cancer. These sites are the colon and rectum, lung, breast, uterus, oral cavity, and non-Hodgkins lymphoma. Many cancers can be prevented by avoiding tobacco, sun exposure, excess dietary fat, and other environmental factors that are known to be carcinogenic. Approximately 30 percent of all deaths due to cancer are related to tobacco use. This number translates into one in six deaths in the United States each year. Diet is suspected to be responsible for 35 percent of deaths due to cancer,[1] and most skin cancers are caused by excessive sun exposure.

Many cancers can be cured if they are found and treated early. In addition to a self breast exam every month, regular cancer checkups, including a mammogram, pap test, and rectal exam are important.

Cancer Facts 1999[2]

The good news is that breast cancer mortality dropped 1.7 percent, and colon and rectum cancer dropped 1.5 percent between the years 1990 and 1995.

The estimated number of new cancers in all sites for women in 1999 was 598,000. The estimated number of deaths for women for cancer in all sites in 1999 was 272,000. The 10 most common cancers of women are breast, lung, colon and rectum, uterus, ovary, non-Hodgkin's lymphomas, melanoma, urinary, pancreas, and thyroid. Breast, lung, and colon and rectum cancers are the most common forms of cancer. These three sites are expected to result in more than 50 percent of all new cancers. Breast cancer is expected to result in 29 percent, or 175,000 new cases of cancer. African-American women have the highest rates of cancer of all women.

Antioxidants and Cancer

Hundreds of studies have been conducted to find a cause for cancer. Assessing cancer risk in relation to micronutrients is difficult. Although no magic fix, or cancer inhibitor, has been identified, some agents have been associated with lower risks. A 1997 review of 53 studies assessed the association of vitamins and minerals with the incidence of cancer. The reviewers found what they called modest evidence of a protective effect of vitamin supplements against cancer. The following are some of their findings:

- The most consistent association was with vitamin E. There was a 50 percent reduction of risk of cancer between users and nonusers.
- Vitamin supplement users had fewer oral pharyngeal cancers than nonusers.
- Three studies found supplementation with vitamin A reduced the risk of breast cancer.
- Vitamin C had an inverse association with bladder cancer.
- Selenium had a strong protective effect on total number of lung and prostate cancers.[3]

The best protection against lung cancer is not to smoke and not be around smoke. However, in a follow-up of NHANES I, vitamin E, vitamin C, and carotenoids may reduce the risk of developing lung cancer. The intake of these nutrients from supplements may be beneficial for those people who have a poor nutritional status. However, the beneficial effects from supplements remain unproven. Daily diets should consist of a variety of fruits and vegetables that provide these nutrients.[4] Other studies have found similar protective associations from eating a diet filled with vegetables and fruits.[5,6]

Human papillomavirus (HPV) shows a significant role in cervical carcinogenesis. Women who tested positive for HPV had decreased concentrations of carotenoids and tocopherols. This is another story of the chicken and the egg: Which came first, low levels of the nutrients, or does the HPV lower serum levels?[7]

Dietary supplementation with vitamin C, tocopherols, and vitamins B6 have been shown to enhance immune function. When the immune system is activated, stress is increased on the antioxidant defenses depleting the supply of antioxidants. For the immune system to work properly, the antioxidants need to be replaced.[8]

Another study showed that a plant-based diet, low in calories from fats, high in fiber, and rich in legumes (especially soybeans), whole grain foods, vegetables, and fruits, reduced the risk of endometrial cancer.[9]

For specific studies reducing the risk of cancer, see individual vitamins and minerals in Section II.

Breast Cancer

Both genetics and environmental factors play a part to increase the risk of breast cancer. The BRCA1 gene was discovered in 1994. Originally, researchers believed that 80 to 90 percent of the women with this gene would develop breast cancer.[10] Now this estimate has been reduced to a risk of 56 percent.[11] Another gene, BRCA2 has been discovered as well. Only 5 to 10 percent of all breast cancers can be contributed to either gene. In women under age 70 with ovarian cancer, 3 to 8 percent have mutations in the BRCA1 gene.[12] Genetic counseling and testing are available for those women who are at high risk of having the gene.

Dietary fat and the use of hormones have been examined to determine their roles in promoting cancer. The studies have proven to be controversial, and the methodology in the studies has been questioned. (See Chapters 25 and 28.) It is difficult to control for the number of variables that exist and for individual differences. These factors make the determination of cause and effect extremely difficult.

It is interesting to compare various countries' lifestyles and their rates of cancer and mortality. The United States has one of the highest rates of breast cancer in the world. Japan has about one-fourth the rate of breast cancer as does the United States and has the longest life expectancy in the world. The two countries have many dietary differences. Traditional Japanese consume about 11 percent of their calories as fat. They generally eat a low-meat, high-fiber, heavily fish-based diet.[13] People in the United States consume about 40 percent of their calories from fat and eat a high-meat, low-fiber diet. Research has shown that women whose diets are high in fiber and low in fat have lower estrogen levels than women whose diets are low in fiber and high in fat. A research project on postmenopausal women found that meat-eating women in Boston had a 300 percent higher serum level of natural estrogen than Asian immigrants living in Hawaii. Estrogen levels were also found to be 30 to 75 percent higher in premenopausal meat-eating women than in Asian immigrants.[14] When Japanese women adopt a western diet similar to that of the United States, their rate of breast cancer increases to that found in the United States.[15] Another study found that women who ate a low-fat, high-carbohydrate diet for two years had reduced density on a mammogram. Large areas of dense breast tissue seen on a mammogram are associated with an increased risk of breast cancer.[16]

However, a longitudinal study, called The Harvard Nurses Health Study, began in 1976. More than 120,000 women were monitored over a decade using successive questionnaires covering multiple areas, including estrogen use, smoking habits, eating habits, and overall health. The results indicated that the risk of breast cancer due to a diet with more than 50 percent fat was no higher than that from a diet with as much as 29 percent fat.[17] Dr. Peter Greenwald, a cancer specialist at the National Institute of Health points out that the nurses study only looked at women whose fat intake was 27 to 50 percent of their total caloric intake. It may be necessary to reduce the amount of fat intake below 20 or 25 percent of total calories to see a reduction in the risk of breast cancer. The nurses study did not look at these lower fat intakes.[18] The Harvard School of Public Health reported, in a 1992 conference, an association between trans-fatty acid intake and breast cancer in the review of 85,000 nurses.[19] Similar results were found in a European study: 6,982 postmenopausal women with primary breast cancer had higher levels of trans-fatty acids in their breast tissue when biopsied.[20] (See Chapter 28 for a discussion of trans-fatty acids.) As if trans-fatty acids were not bad enough now another "nonfood" source called olestra has been developed. It has been shown to inhibit the absorption of beta-carotene and lycopene. These antioxidants are some of the better known protective agents against cancer. (See Chapter 28.) Presently studies are still conflicting as to the association of fat consumption and breast cancer. Studies that focus on a single nutrient cannot always include other interactive effects of our lifestyle. Hopefully The Women's Health Initiative and the Women's Intervention Nutrition Study that are currently underway to assess fat-caloric intake and obesity association will help answer more of these questions.[21]

Recently attention has turned away from fats to another longstanding suspect—estrogen exposure. The length of time spent bathing the breast tissues in a cyclically fluctuating estrogen environment appears to affect the risk of breast cancer. Thus early menarche (first menstruation) and late menopause both have been associated with increased risk. This may be one of the reasons for the disparate rates of breast cancer in the United States and in countries such as China. Presently Chinese women begin to menstruate at the age of 17, just as North American women did 200 years ago. Today women in the United States begin to menstruate at a mean age of 12.5 years. The sustained, high hormonal levels associated with pregnancy, however, appear to be protective against later breast cancer development—so much so that a woman who has her first child at age 20 has half the breast cancer risk of a woman who waits until 30.[22]

Estrogen replacement therapy and hormone replacement therapy cause concern and controversy over the extent of the increased risk of cancer. A Swedish study of 23,244 women found a link between estrogen therapy and breast cancer. The results of the study found that women doubled their risk of breast cancer after using estradiol for a nine-year period. Women who took estradiol with a progestin increased the risk of breast cancer fourfold.

The researchers in the Nurses Health Study found a 35 to 36 percent increase in breast cancer in women who took estrogen compared to those who did not.[23,24] In the 1995 follow-up study, researchers found a 40 percent increased risk of cancer among women 50 to 64 years old who used HRT for five or more years, and a 70 percent increase in risk in women between 65 and 69 years of age.[25]

Others have concluded that women who take estrogen replacement therapy have a 40 percent increased risk of breast cancer over women who have never used estrogen. Women on the birth control pill have a 50 percent increased risk of breast cancer while on the pill. The rates of cancer drop back to baseline once the estrogen is stopped. It is suspected that estrogen may promote the growth of existing tumors rather than initiate the growth.[26]

Still others found that, although women who used estrogen had an increased risk of breast cancer, estrogen users who developed cancer had a 10 to 20 percent lower risk of cancer death than nonusers who developed breast cancer. These findings have been attributed to the fact that women using estrogen are screened more closely and the tumors are found earlier than in nonusers.[27] A 50-year-old woman's risk of breast cancer is approximately 3 percent. By taking estrogen replacement therapy, it increases to 4 percent. Fractures are reduced from 3 percent to approximately 1.5 to 2 percent; the 30 percent risk of cardiac death is reduced to 15 percent.[28]

The use of HRT may promote lesions that predispose women to breast cancer. Women treated with HRT require strict monitoring. In a study of 156 women who had benign breast lesions, 57 of the biopsies revealed that they were predisposed to future breast cancer; 63 percent of those women were being treated with HRT.[29]

In all fairness, even considering the possible increased risk of breast cancer, many authorities still favor treatment with HRT/ERT in view of the fact that it protects against heart disease, which kills 10 times as many women as breast cancer in the United States.

Studies conducted on antioxidants have not been able to find any significant interactions between antioxidant levels and the risk of breast cancer.[30] In a follow-up study of the Netherlands Cohort Study of

62,573 women, beta-carotene, vitamin E, dietary fiber, supplements with vitamin C, and vegetables showed no association with breast cancer risk.[31] Another large study of 34,387 postmenopausal women from Iowa whose diets were assessed by a questionnaire found little association between the intake of vitamin A, C, and E and risk of breast cancer.[32] In a group of 347 women with breast cancer and 374 women without breast cancer, there was no association between antioxidants and hormone-related cancer.[33]

Risks

Breast cancer is increased by oral contraceptive use. However, the increased risk is diminished 10 years after discontinuing use.

Breast cancer risk is increased by younger age of menarche, older age at menopause, and older age of first birth. DDT has been shown to hasten the onset of puberty.

Risk is increased approximately three years following childbirth. Breast feeding may protect against breast cancer.

Tall women may have increased risk of breast cancer.

Women with breast cancer tend to have high bone mass. This could be a result of long-term estrogen exposure.

Women who test positively for the BRCA1 and/or BRCA2 gene have a higher risk of breast cancer.

Family history increases risk. A mother with breast cancer increases the risk two to three times. A mother and a sister with breast cancer increases the risk six times.

Women who have never borne a child or who have had their first full-term pregnancy after age 30 have a two- to three-fold increase risk of breast cancer as compared to women having a full-term pregnancy before age 20.

Studies are still mixed about whether oral birth control raises the risk of breast cancer. However, it looks like women who started taking oral contraceptives at a young age may have a higher risk.

Long-term use of hormone replacement has been associated with increased risk.

Alcohol increases the risk. Intensity of drinking may be an important factor for breast cancer risk. Women who drank five or more grams, about half a drink a day, had a 50 percent increase in breast cancer. The greater the number years of drinking alcohol, the higher the risk of breast cancer.

Obesity beginning and persisting after age 30 is associated with increased risk of postmenopausal breast cancer. Higher body mass was associated with a lower breast cancer incidence in premenopausal women. Women who do not use postmenopausal hormones and have higher body mass have a higher risk.[34] Lean women appear to be at increased risk of premenopausal breast cancer.

Radiation exposure increases breast cancer risk. Exposure to radiation before age 20 increases the risk of later breast cancer. Radiation among women over 40 shows only a modest increased risk.[35]

Reducing the Risk of Breast Cancer

Preventive measures to reduce risk of menopausal breast cancers are best begun before the menopause.

A vegetarian type diet may protect against cancer. Vegetarians generally show lower plasma estradiol levels than nonvegetarians. Animal products contain high levels of fat and organochlorine residues that increase serum levels of estrogen.

Physical activity may protect against breast cancer by influencing body weight and menstrual cycle. Rigorous exercise during adulthood showed great protection.[36]

Soy protein is a source of isoflavones with antiestrogen properties. Genistein, found in soy products, has been shown to inhibit mammary tumors.

Wheat bran reduced estradiol levels in premenopausal women.[37, 38]

Olive oil consumption has been associated with a reduced risk of breast cancer.

Panfrying meats and fish was associated with a decreased risk, whereas stewing and broiling was associated with increased risk. Pickled vegetables increased risk, whereas, fresh vegetables did not.[39]

A study of 5,353 women who were recurrence-free of breast cancer after 5 to 15 years showed that the women who had surgery performed during the luteal phase, days 14 to 23 of the menstrual cycle, had a 5 percent better survival rate when compared to those operated on in the beginning of their cycle.[40]

Fermented milk, such as yogurt with lactobacilli, shows antitumor activity. Women who consume fermented milk products may have a reduced risk of breast cancer.[41]

See Chapter 28 for cancer prevention recommendations by the American Cancer Society, the American Institute of Cancer Research, and the U.S. Department of Human Services. See Section II, individual chapters on the antioxidant nutrients for their associations with reduced cancer risks.

Screening

Mammography sensitivity increases with age. Premenopausal women tend to have denser breast tissue than postmenopausal women. Dense breast tissue is more difficult to read than fatty breast tissue on a mammogram. Mammography may be less accurate for women taking hormone replacement because of increased breast density due to the HRT.

The National Cancer Institute presently recommends mammography every one to two years for women in their 40s at average risk, and every year after 50. A self breast exam, is recommended every month, at the same time in your cycle.

25

Estrogen and Hormone Replacement Therapies

APPROXIMATELY 40 million women of menopausal age live in the United States today. This number is expected to grow to 50 million in the year 2000. Worldwide, it is estimated that more than 300 million women may be menopausal. Currently hormone replacement is the most commonly prescribed medication; approximately 31.7 million prescriptions are written every year in the United States. Yet only 10 to 25 percent of menopausal women take HRT, and only 50 percent of all HRT prescriptions are filled. Less than 40 percent of women who take HRT do so for more than one year. The main reasons women refuse to use HRT are the fear of malignancy, breakthrough bleeding, weight gain, and moodiness. Women generally believe that menopause is a transition in life, not a disease.[1]

Many women today are using alternative or complementary therapies. Some of these include relaxation techniques, massage, herbal medicines, homeopathy, and acupuncture. In a phone survey of 1,539 women, 34 percent reported using at least one complementary therapy in the past year.[2]

Women taking estrogen replacement therapy (ERT) or hormone replacement therapy (HRT), a combination of estrogen and a progestogen, need to know and understand the unresolved issues and concerns about these treatments. ERT and HRT are relatively new therapies, and the research studies are incomplete. Never before has such a large proportion of aging women taken drugs to prolong a hormonal state similar to that of younger women. Both benefits and risks accompany this type of therapy. Some of the consequences may be yet unknown.[3]

Listed below are a sampling of recommendations made by physicians and researchers:

- Hormone therapy should be given to premenopausal women who have had a hysterectomy, have coronary heart disease, or are at high risk for coronary heart disease.[4] Yet this is still disputed.

- Short-term therapy with a gradual withdrawal is beneficial for menopausal problems. Long-term therapy, a minimum 10 years, or life-long therapy may be necessary for cardiac and bone health. The effects of HRT wear off within a few years of discontinuation.

- Hormone therapy should be recommended for women who have had a hysterectomy, have had bilateral oophorectomies, have coronary heart disease, or are at risk for coronary heart disease. However, the benefits of HRT are not clearly understood and the increased risk of breast cancer is a concern. More research is needed.[5]

- Hormone therapy is clearly indicated for women who have lost their ovaries before age 40, have a strong history of osteoporosis, or have a history of long-term steroid use.[6]

Women have different physical and emotional needs and risks. Each woman needs to be aware of the pros and cons of ERT/HRT and must make a personal decision depending on her particular needs. It is a difficult, confusing decision because of the lack of information about the long-term effects and because of the range of opinion concerning treatments. Various authorities have widely divergent opinions concerning the use of ERT/HRT. The National Women's Health Network has opposed the widespread treatment of healthy women with ERT/HRT to prevent diseases they may never get. It is still unclear whether the benefits of the HRT outweigh the risks.[7, 8]

The U.S. FDA has approved Premarin[9] estrogen therapy for hot flashes, atrophic vaginitis (thinning and drying changes), osteoporosis, low estrogen states due to removal or failure of the ovaries, uterine bleeding due to hormonal imbalance, and for palliation (alleviation of symptoms rather than cure) in cases of advanced breast cancer.[10, 11] In

1990 the FDA's Fertility and Maternal Health Drugs Advisory Committee judged that replacement therapy with Premarin may have value in reducing women's risks of heart and blood vessel diseases. Note that although several different estrogen preparations are used in the United States, their effects are not identical and neither are their indicated uses.

Estrogen Therapy (ERT)

Contraindications of ERT

- Active cancer of the breast, uterus, or ovary or history of recent cancer (less than five years) of the breast, uterus, or ovary.
- Liver disease including hepatitis.
- Undiagnosed vaginal bleeding.
- Pregnancy (may cause birth defects).
- Active deep vein thrombophlebitis.
- Uncontrolled high blood pressure.

Advantages of ERT

- Eliminates hot flashes and night sweats.
- Reduces loss of calcium from the bones, lowering the risk of osteoporosis.
- Prevents drying and shrinking of vaginal and urinary tract tissues.
- Reduces heart disease, increases the production of HDL (good) cholesterol, and decreases the level of LDL (bad) cholesterol.
- May reduce the risk of colorectal cancer.
- May improve symptoms of Alzheimer's disease.

Disadvantages of ERT

- Estrogen unopposed by progesterone increases risk of endometrial cancer 5- to 14-fold in women who have uteri. The addition of progesterone reduces this risk.

- May increase the risk of breast cancer by 30 to 60 percent.[12] This is still a controversial issue.

Hormone Replacement Therapy (HRT)

Advantages of HRT

- Reduces loss of calcium from the bones, lowering the risk of osteoporosis.[13, 14]
- Eliminates hot flashes and night sweats.
- Prevents drying and shrinking of vaginal and urinary tract tissues.
- Reduces mood swings.

Note: There is a distinct difference between synthetic progestogens and natural progesterone. Natural progesterone is identical to the progesterone produced in a woman's body. Synthetic progestogens are similar but not identical. As a result more side effects may exist with the synthetic progestogens. (See Chapter 32.)

Disadvantages of HRT

- Studies are still inconclusive concerning the affects of progestins and heart disease. However, natural progesterones and nonandrogenic progestins do not affect the blood lipids as much as progestin.[15]
- HRT may cause bloating, cramping, breast tenderness, nausea, depression.
- It may cause uterine bleeding and uterine fibroids.
- It increases risk of breast cancer. The risk of breast cancer is moderately increased after 10 or more years of HRT.[16]
- HRT may promote lesions that predispose women to breast cancer. Women treated with HRT require strict monitoring. In a study of 156 women who had benign breast lesions, 57 of the biopsies revealed that they were predisposed to future breast cancer; 63 percent of those women were being treated with HRT.[17]

A Problem ERT/HRT Can't Eliminate

Aging and skin wrinkling is not eliminated by ERT/HRT. But estrogen supplementation does make the skin a little plumper and less dry due to increased collagen production.[18]

Pills, Patches, Injections, and Creams

Estrogen can be taken by mouth in pill form. It enters the body, is absorbed through the digestive tract and processed by the liver, then enters the bloodstream.

Skin patches allow low, steady doses of the hormone to enter the bloodstream directly, bypassing the liver, until it is introduced into the body's circulatory system. This avoids much trouble with liver and gallbladder problems. However, 20 percent of women will develop rashes from the patch application, which is placed on the abdomen or hip twice a week. Patches do help with menopausal complaints, but long-term studies are needed to determine the effects on heart disease, osteoporosis, and breast cancer.

Injection of estrogen directly under the skin allows a slow absorption into the blood without having to go through the stomach or liver first. These injections are usually given by a physician every three to four weeks.

Vaginal estrogen creams can be applied once or twice a week to help relieve vaginal dryness or urinary problems. When the estrogen dosage is very low, little estrogen enters the bloodstream, lessening both the risks and benefits of estrogen to the body's tissues. However, higher dosages of vaginal estrogens will be absorbed well and have more pronounced systemic effects.

Progestin creams have also been used to eliminate problems associated with menopause and PMS. The application depends on the individual woman and problem. Progestogen therapy is useful in women who cannot take estrogen or who have developed side effects to estrogens.

Natural progesterone cream has been shown to eliminate most menopausal complaints without side effects. In cream form the progesterone is biologically available. Progesterone taken orally is transported to the liver, metabolized, and excreted in bile and is therefore not as biologically available. To assess progesterone levels, saliva tests are more useful than blood serum tests. This is because progesterone is fat soluable, and almost all the circulating progesterone measured in serum is inactive and bound to protein. Saliva tests do a better job of measuring the minute amounts of active, unbound hormone. These tests are available without a doctor's prescription.

Androgen cream may be effective in preventing vaginal dryness. Testosterone creams may increase a woman's libido after a hysterectomy. However, there may be permanent masculizing effects from its use, such as a deepened voice, increased facial hair, and an enlarged clitoris.[19]

Summary

- The use of ERT/HRT is an individualized decision. Be aware of the facts and risks before making a decision.

- ERT is protective against cardiac disease, the number one killer of women over 50. One study suggests that ERT reduces the risk of cardiovascular disease by 40 to 60 percent.[20] However, generally ERT was only given to healthy women, which may account for reduced incidences of heart attack rates with estrogen users.[21] ERT increases the risk of breast cancer.

- Fewer studies have been conducted comparing HRT and cardiac diseases than with ERT. Some studies have conflicting results regarding the advantages. HRT may also raise the rate of breast cancer more than ERT.

- Some women find relief from hot flashes and vaginal and urinary tract problems by taking ERT/HRT for a short time and then discontinuing the treatment gradually.[22] Many women use the treatment for less than one year for menopausal complaints.

- Women with uteri should take progesterone along with their estrogen to prevent endometrial cancer. There is a 5- to 14-fold increase of cancer reported with ERT alone.

• Both ERT and HRT reduce the risk of osteoporosis by reducing bone loss. The time necessary for using hormones as a prevention for osteoporosis is unknown. Some researchers state that the necessary treatment period may be 6 years, some say 10 years, and some say lifetime treatment. A bone density test can be done to see if you need ERT/HRT for this purpose.

• ERT is generally recommended for premenopausal women who have had oophorectomies. However, natural progesterone is sometimes supplemented.

• It appears that the longer a women is on ERT/HRT, the greater the risk of breast cancer, especially for those women who are genetically predisposed. (See alternatives to ERT/HRT, Chapter 31.)

26

Exercise

As we age, fat mass increases and muscle mass decreases. Bone density declines as well. Generally, women who have little muscle development also have a subnormal amount of bone.[1] However, the situation is not hopeless. We can help our bodies by exercising. A study that examined muscle strength and aging found that people up to age 96 were able to increase their muscle size and strength by up to 200 percent.[2] Research shows that for overall good health, specifically our hearts and bones, both aerobic and weight-bearing exercises are essential. Following are some benefits of exercise:

- Helps to prevent heart disease. Lack of exercise has been established as a risk factor for heart disease. A sedentary lifestyle increases the risk of a heart attack by almost two times.[3] The data from more than 40 studies indicated that coronary artery heart disease is 1.9 times more likely to occur in inactive people.[4]

- Helps blood vessels transport blood and oxygen to every cell in the body.

- Increases bone strength and helps prevent osteoporosis. (See Chapter 23.)

- Stimulates the ovaries and adrenal glands to produce estrogen.

- Improves lung function and increases efficiency of oxygen use in tissues.

- Controls weight.
- Relieves tension.
- Controls high blood pressure.
- May help control cigarette smoking.
- Increases energy levels and resistance to fatigue.
- Improves ability to sleep.
- Increases flexibility.

The American Heart Association states that exercises should be done vigorously for 30 to 60 minutes three to four times a week at the target heart rate zone. Exercises should be rhythmic and repetitive, involve motion and the use of large muscles, and work the circulatory system.[5] (See the following table for the target maximum heart rate zone.[6])

Age (Years)	Target Heart Rate Zone (50–75% of maximum in beats/minute)	Average Maximum Heart Rate (100% in beats/minute)
20	100–150	200
25	98–146	195
30	95–142	190
35	93–138	185
40	90–135	180
45	88–131	175
50	85–127	170
55	83–123	165
60	80–120	160
65	78–116	155
70	75–113	150

Source: Reproduced with permission. ©"Exercise Diary," 1993–1996. Copyright American Heart Association.

To check your heart rate, during and after exercising, place your first two fingers on your carotid arteries, the blood vessels in your neck on either side of the Adam's apple. Or you can check your pulse on the inside of your wrist just below the thumb. Count the pulses for 10 seconds and multiply that number by six. Check the number against the chart. If the number is too low, put a little more effort in the exercise. If the number is too high, slow down a little bit. When the pulse rate is too high, the effect is anaerobic. The body cannot keep up with the demand for oxygen, and the maximum benefits of exercising cannot be realized. One general rule is that while you are exercising you should always be able to talk and carry on a conversation.

It may be important to check with a doctor before you begin exercising or to help you find an appropriate exercise program, especially if you have a history of heart disease or high blood pressure, or are on medication. After choosing the activity, build endurance slowly over a few weeks. Start the exercise with a warm-up period, including stretching. After exercising, end with a cool-down period, also including stretching. Listen to your body. If something causes pain, stop! Check with a physician if you have any pain or pressure in the left- or mid-chest area, left neck, left shoulder, or arm, or if you experience light-headedness, cold sweats, pallor, or fainting. These may be signs of heart problems.

Kegel Exercises

Women also have a specific need to exercise the pelvic area. These exercises can be made a part of a daily routine. They can be done while doing other exercises, such as abdominal exercises, or even while sitting in the car.

During the late 1940s, Dr. Arnold Kegel, a UCLA surgeon, designed a special set of exercises for women who complained of urinary incontinence. Leaking urine can happen gradually throughout the day or as a result of a sneeze, cough, or laughter. The exercises Dr. Kegel developed proved to be surprisingly effective in restoring bladder control. The exercises focus on strengthening the pubococcygeal muscle, which supports the bladder and the urethra.[7,8] Properly developed, this muscle can stop the flow of urine in midstream, control bowel movements, and adds to increased sexual satisfaction. During sexual activity, it contracts rhythmically with orgasm.

Dr. Kegel's first 500 cases had a 84 percent rate of restoration of urinary continence during the exercise program. The study included some women in their 80s who found the exercises effective even though surgery had not corrected their problems.[9]

Learning and performing these exercises are not difficult, but the target muscles must first be identified in order to know what to strengthen. Many adult women do not know how to identify these muscles. One way to accustom yourself to the feeling of contracting the pubococcygeal muscle is to stop the flow of urine when going to the bathroom. Another way is to insert one or two fingers into the vagina and squeeze the finger with the inner muscles. Soon you will be able to consciously contract the muscle to exercise and strengthen it.

The following technique, an easy way to learn how to do the exercises, can be done anywhere.

1. Lie on your back on the floor or on a firm surface. Use a mat or rug to rest on.

2. Draw up the pelvic floor, the target muscles, and squeeze. Hold for three seconds and then relax. Repeat this five times.

3. Tighten the muscles slowly up toward the abdomen as high as possible and then slowly release them back down. A number of authors have compared the muscles to an elevator in a building that has five floors. At each elevator stop, hold the muscles tight, count to five, and move up to the next floor. Continue all the way up to the fifth floor, or as high as the muscles will allow, and then relax the muscles at each floor on the way down. Repeat the series five times.

4. Pretend to draw water into and up the vagina. Repeat this five times.[10, 11]

A few other devices may also help control incontinence:

- A tampon inserted before exercise.

- A urethral patch, which is a foam patch attached with a jelly adhesive to the urethral opening. It is removed to go to the bathroom and then reapplied.

- A urethral plug, which is a small plastic tube with a balloon that blocks urination. Use once and replace.

- A pessary, which is similar to a diaphragm and inserted into the vagina to support the bladder.

- Collagen injection into the surrounding areas of the vulva.
- Surgery and drugs.[12]

Diet and Exercise

Reseachers who have looked at the effect of vitamins and minerals on exercising performance have concluded that it is critical to maintain an adequate diet to perform one's best, and that marginal vitamin and mineral intakes through an inadequate diet result in poor athletic performance.[13] In a review of the subject, another researcher concluded that poor diets, not exercise, are probably the main reason for most mineral deficiencies in athletes.[14] Exceptions seem to be iron and zinc, which may well be depleted by heavy exercise.[15, 16, 17] Supplementation may be important for good health, but there was little evidence that it helped athletic performance. On the other hand, numerous studies can point to significant biochemical differences in exercising individuals who take antioxidants such as beta-carotene, vitamin E, and vitamin C. These vitamins do apparently protect against oxidative damage to tissue that is otherwise seen during or after heavy exercise.[18, 19] Furthermore, recent data suggest that eating carbohydrates prior to and even during exercise is beneficial in increasing endurance[20] and in sparing the breakdown of muscle protein.

Earlier recommendations for protein intake in athletes were likely too low. As much as 5 to 6 percent of the calories burned during exercise come from metabolizing muscle tissue. This translates into an increased need for dietary protein during athletic training.[21, 22]

Research indicates that there are not any magic formulas to enhance exercise performance. But here are a few helpful tips:

- Vegetarian athletes need to be especially aware of the difficulties of obtaining protein, iron, zinc, calcium, and vitamin B_{12} from a purely vegetarian diet,[23] and may need to consider broadening their diets or taking supplements.

- Human studies on exercise support dietary supplementation of antioxidant vitamins. They have favorable effects on lipid peroxidation after exercise. Since free-radical production increases during exercise, antioxidants play a protective role in exercise-induced muscle damage. Vitamin E is consumed by muscles and other tissues during increased physical activity.[24]

- Thiamine requirements are dependent on carbohydrate intake. This may be important since some athletes load carbohydrates.[25]

- The requirements of riboflavin are possibly higher in women athletes.[26]

- Vitamin C is thought to improve heat acclimatization in athletes.[27]

- Vitamin E may be helpful when exercising in high altitudes.[28, 29] There is also evidence that supplementation protects against muscle damage during exercise and increases the rate of rebuilding muscle tissue, especially in older individuals.[30, 31]

- Although chromium picolinate has been touted as a natural steroid, I could not find such data to back the antidotal claims. However, chromium is known to significantly influence insulin metabolism and thus may also affect the metabolism of fats and muscle protein as well. (See Chapter 12.)

- Women athletes tend to be at risk for low iron levels because of low iron intakes and menstrual loss. Long-distance runners, both male and female, are also at risk for low iron levels.[32]

- Magnesium levels have been shown to be low after exercising, but so far no need for supplementation has been established.[33]

- Zinc levels are generally found to be low in athletes but supplementation has not been shown to affect strenuous activity.[34]

Athletes with low caloric intakes need to eat food high in calcium, zinc, magnesium, B_{12}, and iron. On the other hand, athletes who have high caloric intakes should eat foods high in B vitamins.[35] One authority recommends that the optimal diet for athletes should have the following proportions: 60 to 75 percent of calories in carbohydrates, 15 to 20 percent of calories from protein, and no more than 20 to 30 percent of calories from fats.[36]

The American and Canadian Dietetic Associations currently recommend protein intakes of 1.0 to 1.5 grams per kilogram body weight for training athletes, as opposed to the RDA of 0.8 grams per kilogram.[37]

Optimizing Aerobic Exercise Intensity

Robert Greenwell, M.D., sports medicine and cardiac rehabilitation

I HAVE BEEN a member of The American College of Sports Medicine (ACSM) since 1968 and elected to fellowship (with voting and office holding privileges) in 1976. In 1989 I attended the ACSM position stand committee meeting where the proposed revision of the ACSM Official Position on exercise prescription was to be discussed. After the discussion started, I requested a copy of the document being considered for approval by the college. I was told that "nobody is allowed to see these documents, other than the officials, until after they are finalized and published." Therefore, no open dialogue was allowed regarding the content of this guideline before it was published as a document that was approved by ACSM. Those who read these documents are led to believe that the college members evaluated this matter and decided that this was the best possible answer to exercise prescription development. Even the fellows (voting members) of the ACSM were not allowed to have access to the proposed guidelines until after they had been proclaimed accepted and authorized by the few individuals who were appointed to speak for the entire ACSM. Scientific evaluation was compromised. The 1990 official paper on exercise prescriptions stated that "the important factor is to design a program for the individual to provide the proper amount of physical activity to attain maximum benefit at the lowest risk."

In 1992 a few individuals represented the ACSM in a meeting with the Center for Disease Control (CDC) in Atlanta. They accepted the goal of trying to get more people to do some exercise as recommended. Instead of attempting to provide guidelines for helping people to do the best possible in becoming as healthy as possible, they chose the goal of getting the percentage of people following the recommendations to increase. They decided this goal could best be approached by telling people they did not need to change their exercise habits more than a minimal amount. They may have caused more people to follow their guidelines, but they were unable to provide any data to verify that those who followed their guidance would improve their health or functional capacity significantly. They chose a goal that would provide little, if any, benefit rather than accepting the responsibility of trying to provide optimum guidance on how people could obtain the maximum benefit possible, safely. This may have influenced more people to change their habits, but it is unlikely that it changed anyone's health or functional capacity significantly. They did neglect those who were the most interested in helping themselves to become as healthy as possible. Likewise the American Heart Association, the U.S. Department of Health and Human Services, The National Heart Lung and Blood Institute, the Public Health Service Agency for Health Care Policy and Research, the American College of Cardiology, and the U.S. Surgeon General's Office are publishing guidelines that do not provide optimum guidance, but rather maximum compliance.

ACSM's original guideline was published in 1978. It was slightly modified (regarding intensity of training) in 1990. The majority of people are advised to determine the exercise intensity from a calculation of their predicted maximum heart rate. These guidelines are being taught by approximately 450,000 counselors and teachers. They usually advise people to base the results on a calculation of subtracting their age from the magic number 220 to decide their maximum pulse rate. This has been shown to be correct within the unacceptable range of + or – 35 percent. For example, I have measured the maximum pulse rate of a 16-year-old at 186 (instead of 204) and a 35-year-old man at 220 (instead of 185).

Some people injure themselves or even suffer fatal results from overexercise because of inadequate guidance. Many more underexercise and suffer disuse deterioration because they do not challenge their capabilities adequately enough to convince Mother Nature that they will use the capabilities if she will provide them. She tends to grant improvements only if she sees that what she has previously provided is being used.

I have composed this article to guide those who would like to become, and remain, as healthy as possible. Since health is measured by how well the tissues perform the tasks for which they were designed, the functional capacity of an organ or cell indicates the level of health. The healthiest is the most functional. Many authoritative figures have claimed that health benefits can be attained from exercise programs that do not appreciably affect performance (functional capacity). But since health is measured by function, health is not separable from function. Ergo, if health is improved, so must function.

The best of health *is* like self-respect: You must earn it!

People should be most concerned about the health of their hearts and blood vessels. Disease of blood vessels causes more deaths than all other causes combined, including cancers, accidents, infections, and homicide. There has been a trend toward focusing only on the large blood vessels of the body, in part because these large vessels can be treated surgically. Most programs ignore the small blood vessels because they cannot be treated surgically. However, the small vessels are required to deliver oxygen to the tissues, and they can be improved with proper exercise and medication. Due to the physical laws of diffusion, a small change in the density of the capillary bed results in a large change in tissue oxygenation. For example, a 20 percent increase in capillary density actually doubles oxygen delivery capacity. But blood going through a large, surgically treatable artery doesn't improve oxygen delivery if it doesn't improve the blood flow through the capillaries. Programs, such as exercise, that have been shown to improve the small blood vessels can also improve the large vessels and reverse the arteriosclerotic disease process. Surgery does not affect this disease process. Most of what you require for optimal health can only be controlled, or contributed, by you.

It is necessary to determine the intensity of exercise that will produce the maximum benefits possible for each person. Before explaining the procedures for this determination, some of the basic biological principles involved should be brought to mind:

- The health of any cell, organ, or organism is best determined by its capacity for performing the functions it was created to perform. If a cell performs well the functions it was designed by nature to perform, then it is in good health.

- Optimal health treatment (e.g., medical) is the treatment that is most likely to return the affected tissue's functions as near to optimum as possible.

- The energy that enables the cells of the body to stay alive and perform any function is derived almost entirely from the high-energy molecule, adenosine-tri-phosphate (ATP). Cells cannot directly use the energy in fats, sugars, etc., but must first break these molecules down to generate ATP, which they can then use to fuel cellular processes. This is analogous to our common experience with gasoline in our cars: We can use money to buy gas, but our cars won't run on money, only gas.

- Each cell must produce all its own ATP since ATP cannot be transported out of, or into, intact cells.

- A cell cannot maintain functions for extended periods of time at a rate that requires consuming ATP (energy) more rapidly than it can produce ATP. Therefore, the maximum rate of ATP production usually determines the maximum, continuous, functional capacity of each cell that is being provided with normal nutrients. The maximum oxygen delivery rate to a cell may be one of the factors limiting the cell's ATP production rate. When adequate oxygen is delivered, other factors such as intracellular enzyme activity can limit how fast the oxygen can be utilized in producing ATP. The enzymes referred to here utilize oxygen and products derived from fats and carbohydrates to produce ATP. Oxygen delivery, per se, can be the critical event, but how this delivery affects the ATP production rate is the ultimate decisive event.

- The most likely source of the stimuli that increase oxygen delivery to the tissues of the body is from within cells that are capable of using oxygen more rapidly and are being called on to produce ATP more rapidly. For example, when muscle cells go from resting activity to performing work, they will stimulate the processes that improve the oxygen delivery to the working muscles.

- Each cell will attempt to maintain a certain quantity of ATP even though this effort may lead to self-destruction of the cell. Consequently each cell will attempt to produce ATP as rapidly as it uses ATP—with or without adequate oxygen delivery.

People who plan to increase their exercise habits to a greater intensity than they have usually been doing should first be evaluated to determine their maximum safe exercise intensity and the pulse rate at that intensity. Those over age 40, and those with possible heart problems, should have their electrocardiograms monitored continuously during this evaluation. This is to verify that their hearts can safely tolerate the aerobic exercise that their skeletal muscles can tolerate.

People with Heart Risk

People whose heart shows signs that it may not be able to tolerate the aerobic activity that the skeletal muscles can tolerate should be monitored continuously by electrocardiogram during their exercise training episodes. This should be done regularly until the heart metabolism limit becomes greater than the working skeletal muscle tissues' metabolism. For training purposes, maximum heart rate is defined as three to four beats per minute less than the rate was when the electrocardiogram showed signs of impending danger during the initial test. Each week these people should be allowed to exercise at a slightly higher pulse rate if they do not show electrocardiogram signs of myocardial deficiency (either functional or metabolic).

People Without Heart Risk

Those not limited by heart deficiency who wish to safely gain the most benefit possible from the time they are going to spend on aerobic exercise should determine maximum or near maximum heart rate by exercising at their top capacity for a few minutes, then taking their pulse.

Running a few 100-yard dashes at full speed will do fine. So will treadmill exercise pushed to the point where heart rate will not increase any further.

Now that maximum heart rate has been determined by one of the above methods, follow the steps outlined:

1. Warm up by stretching and walking at a moderate pace for approximately 5 to 10 minutes.

2. Then increase the work rate, pace, or exercise intensity to a continuous rate that causes the pulse to reach about 75 percent of the previously demonstrated maximum rate.

3. Continuously (or at least every two minutes) monitor the pulse rate while maintaining the steady intensity (pace) for at least 20 minutes, if the pulse rate does not start increasing greatly above this 75 percent of maximum. If the pulse rate rapidly increases more than five per minute above 75 percent of maximum, the exercise is too intense. You need to decrease the intensity, or pace slightly so that the pulse rate will stabilize and remain stable at a constant exercise intensity.

4. If the pulse rate starts increasing after 10 minutes, you should decrease the pace much more than you would if the pulse starts increasing after 15 minutes. The earlier increase after 10 minutes indicates that the associated pulse rate and pace are extremely excessive.

5. If 75 percent of maximum is excessive as in (4), try a pace that causes the pulse to be maintained at 70 percent of maximum on the next day.

6. Each day thereafter decrease the pace (intensity) or increase it until you identify the fastest pace that causes the pulse rate to rise during the beginning of the training pace and remain reasonably stable for the rest of the 20 to 30 minutes of steady intensity exercise before cooling down.

7. If on the first exercise day the pulse rate remained stable at the pace that maintained the pulse rate at 75 percent of your maximum pulse rate, you should increase the pace so that the pulse rate reaches 80 percent of maximum on the next exercise day.

8. The pace should then be adjusted each day until you identify the fastest pace that will allow the pulse rate to rise during the beginning moments and then remain reasonably stable for the rest of the 20 to 30 minutes of steady exercise before cooling down. This pulse rate will be very close to your maximum steady state pulse rate (MSSPR) for most activities.

9. After the MSSPR has been identified, the only factors that need monitoring during the next year or two is the pulse rate and the duration of the training episodes (20 to 30 minutes). This pulse rate can then be used as a guide for adjusting the pace under variable conditions, such as variable terrain, temperature, or humidity.

10. It will be easiest to determine a person's MSSPR if the exercise episodes are conducted with exercise apparatus that can be adjusted so that the intensity of exercise can be uniform during the test episodes. Machines such as a motorized treadmill, stationary bicycle ergometer, or stationary rowing ergometer will be helpful in maintaining constant test exercise intensity.

After you have verified your MSSPR by the previously described procedure, you will be able to maintain a reasonably constant intensity of exercise by maintaining this pulse rate. If you are walking, jogging, or bicycling on non-level terrain, you should adjust your speed so that the pulse remains near your maximum steady-state rate under these variable conditions during exercise training. The same is true for exercising in high humidity and temperatures, running against a stiff breeze, etc. It is a good guide to use for determining whether you are doing the best you can for improving the heart, blood vessels, and aerobic functional capacity of the tissues being affected by exercise. This procedure will also keep you from exercising at an intensity that is excessive for any significant period of time, which may be unhealthy.

The functions of the muscles, tendons, bones, and ligaments should also be challenged and encouraged to improve maximally (but not beyond their capability) for performing their intended functions better. The heart, lungs, blood vessels, and many other oxygen delivery processes are stimulated by the muscles to improve. If the exercise causes the temperature of the other tissues to also increase, it will be stimulating them to become capable of producing ATP (energy) more rapidly than at rest. After any tissue becomes capable of producing ATP more rapidly, the tissue will be capable of functioning at a higher work rate. For example, if a brain cell can produce energy more rapidly, it can produce thought processes more rapidly, and perhaps more accurately. This may be the reason why studies have shown that people who routinely exercise properly demonstrate better brain function than when they don't routinely exercise properly.

The following graphs are provided to assist you in depicting the events involved in the determination of the best aerobic training intensity of a person.

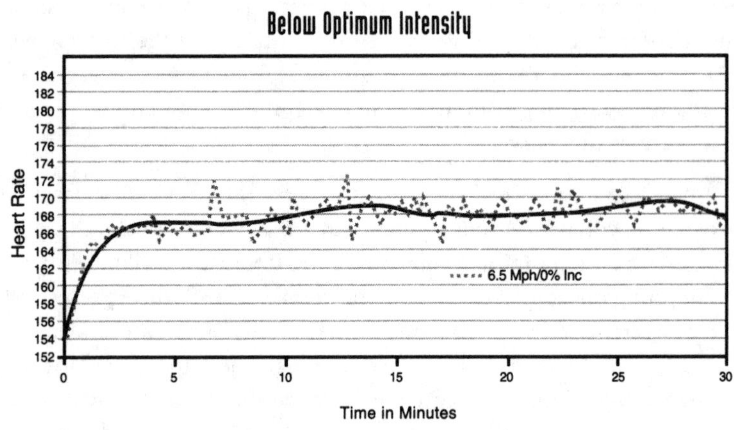

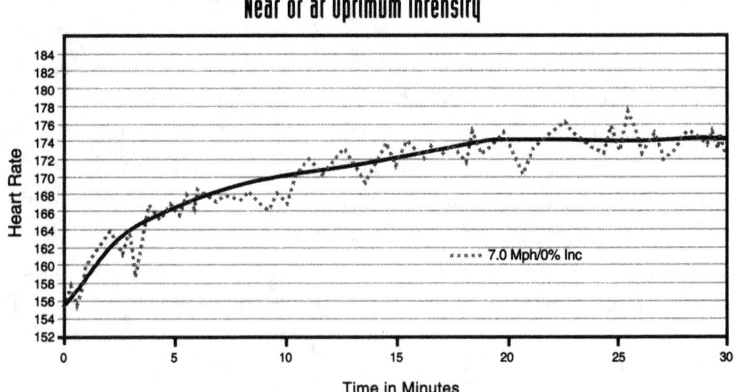

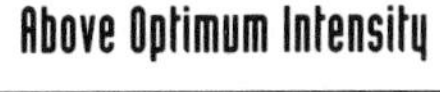

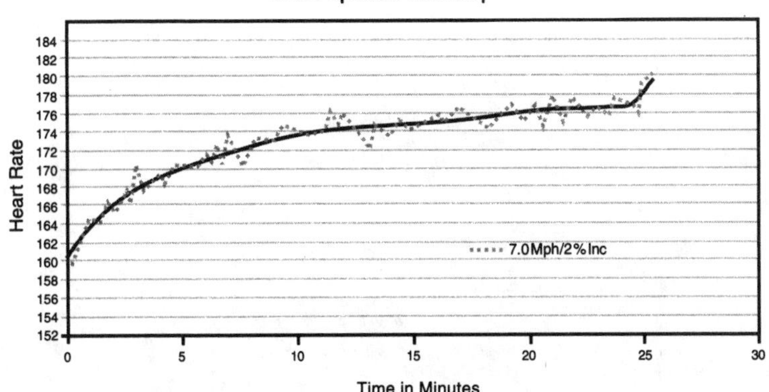

True Maximum

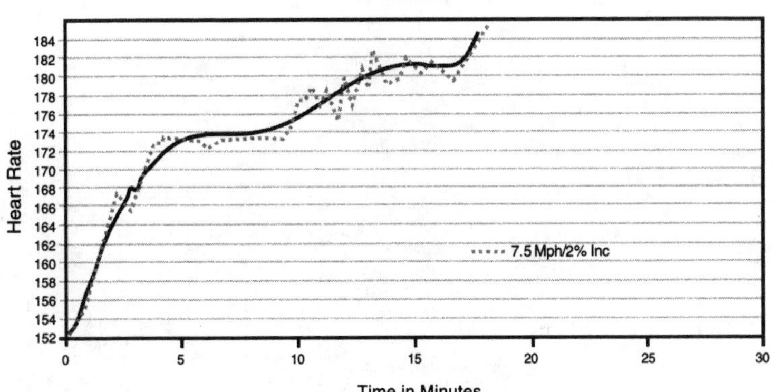

After 6 Months Training at 174 BPM

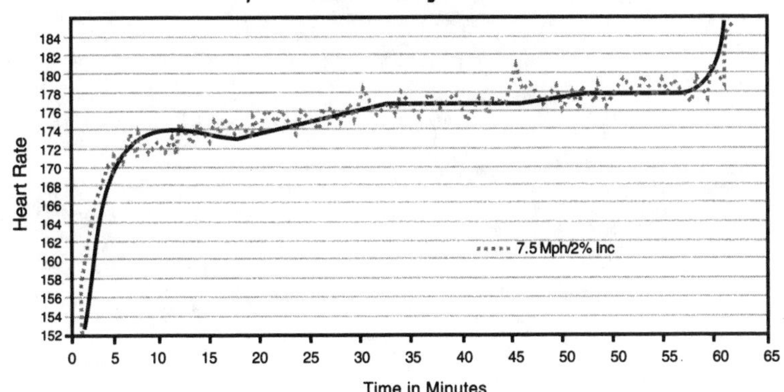

27

Fish Oils

PRIMARY FUNCTIONS

May reduce risk of heart disease
May reduce risk of atherosclerosis
May lower blood pressure
May lower cholesterol
May have positive effects on Crohn's disease; psoriasis; and renal, rheumatic, and gastrointestinal disorders.

FISH OILS—OMEGA-3 fatty acids, or n-3 fatty acids—have been purported to reduce the risk of coronary artery heart disease in a number of different ways: They have been shown to lower cholesterol and triglyceride levels, reduce the stickiness of blood platelets, and increase platelet survival. Small amounts of fish in the diet also provide retinol, selenium, vitamin D, and taurine.[1]

Fish oil has been shown to suppress production of an agent that causes smooth muscle cell growth in the lining of arteries, which may decrease a tendency to form atherosclerotic plaques.[2] Men given fish oil therapy seven days before coronary angioplasty (dilation) and for six months following have shown less than one-half the rate of reblockage than controls did.[3] Restenosis, or reblockage, of the coronary arteries after angioplasty is a major problem, often requiring repeat angioplasty or a bypass operation.

Another study looked at men and women with large artery atherosclerosis. The subjects were supplemented with low doses of omega-3 fatty acids (4 teaspoons of cod liver oil per day). The results indicated that they had prolonged platelet survival times by more than 20 percent. This likely represents a decrease in clotting tendency, which may translate into a decreased chance of heart attack.[4]

Reasearchers have suggested that some polyunsaturated fats can lower blood pressure. One study conducted to determine the effects of n-3 polyunsaturated fats (fish oil) and n-6 polyunsaturated fats (safflower oil) on blood pressure administered different combinations of the fats to men with mild essential hypertension. The results of the study indicated that high levels of fish oils are effective whereas safflower oil is not. However, the researchers were concerned about the safety of high doses of fish oils.[5] A later review indicated that fish oils may be most helpful in persons with hypertension, atherosclerosis, or high cholesterol but showed little effect on the blood pressure of normal individuals.[6]

Fish oils are known to lower levels of plasma triglycerides, but have variously been shown to raise, lower, or have no significant effect on cholesterol levels. These diverse effects may depend on whether the fish oils are replacing or just supplementing animal fats in the diet.[7]

Greenland Eskimos' very low death rate from coronary heart disease has been ascribed to their diets being high in fish. Studies have compared the effects of diets both rich and poor in fish consumption. One sampled 852 middle-aged Dutchmen who began the study without heart disease. In a 20-year follow-up, 78 men had died from heart disease. A 50 percent reduction of mortality due to heart disease occured in the men who consumed at least 30 g of fish a day. The researchers concluded that eating fish one to two times a week may have a preventive value against heart disease.[8] Another 30-year study of 1,822 men showed an inverse association between fish consumption and death from coronary heart disease, especially nonsudden death from myocardial infarction.[9] Some researchers hypothesized that because of the positive effects fish oil has on lipids, it may also help individuals with rheumatoid arthritis, Crohn's disease, and psoriasis, as well as renal, rheumatic, and gastrointestinal diseases.[10, 11, 12]

Try adding some garlic to that fish! The combination has been shown to reduce heart disease, and garlic alone has been shown to reduce triglyceride levels. The combination of fish oil (1,800 mg EPA plus 1,200 mg of docosahexanoic acid) and garlic (1,200 mg of garlic powder) for one month had positive effects on lowering cholesterol and triglycerides.[13]

No specific RDA recommendation has been given. The previously mentioned study supports eating fish one to two times a week. However, a supplemental capsule of fish oil, sold as eicosapentaenoic acid (EPA) generally in doses of 200 or 500 mg is available.

Liver and fish liver oils contain large amounts of vitamin A, which may cause toxicity. (See Chapter 3.) High intakes of fish oils may increase lipid peroxidation in tissues. The increased need for concomitant antioxidants such as vitamin E to counter this effect is unknown at this time.[14]

28

Food

Written with Nan Jensen, R.D., L.D., and Phil Hanna

REMEMBER THE old adage, "You are what you eat!"? That statement holds more meaning today than ever before. Americans are obsessed with food. Food is good conversation, it's fashionable, and some would say, "To die for." Unfortunately that is exactly what some diets are doing to us. This chapter will discuss food and its effect on our lives. Hopefully, after you have digested this chapter, you will be better able to make better choices about what you eat and how you shop.

Poor diet contributes to many diseases. It has been shown to promote cancer, coronary heart disease, osteoporosis, stroke, obesity, and diabetes mellitus. A good diet, on the other hand, is one of the major foundations of good health.

Many different health and governmental organizations have recommendations for a "good" diet. Generally, these guidelines are similar. They all agree that it is important to maintain a healthy body weight, eat a wide variety of foods from all the major food groups, and to imbibe no more than one or two drinks of alcohol per day, if at all. Most recommendations include a reduction of fats to less than 30 percent of the total calories consumed. Less than 10 percent of dietary fats should be saturated fats. Most organizations agree that there should be an increase in both fiber and carbohydrate foods. Cholesterol intake should be no greater than 250 to 300 mg per day. Recommendations vary on sodium. Most say sodium consumption should be less than 2,400 mg per day.

Guidelines

Following are guidelines from different health agencies. Their similarities are obvious after perusing the lists.

The DASH Diet

The Dietary Approach to Stop Hypertension, or DASH diet, is the result of a multicenter study done by the National Heart, Lung, and Blood Institute. The diet significantly lowered both systolic and diastolic blood pressure, especially for people with hypertension.[1, 2] The DASH eating plan as shown below is based on 2,000 calories a day.[3]

Food Group	Daily Servings (except as noted)	Serving Sizes	Examples
Grains and Grain Products	7–8	1 slice bread; ½ cup dry cereal; ½ cup cooked rice, pasta, or cereal	whole grain breads, English muffin, pita bread, cereals, grits, bagel, oatmeal, crackers, unsalted pretzels, popcorn
Vegetables	4–5	1 cup raw leafy vegetable; ½ cup cooked vegetable; 6 oz. vegetable juice	tomatoes, potatoes, carrots, green peas, squash, brocoli, turnip greens, collards, kale, spinach, artichokes, green beans, lima beans, sweet potatoes
Fruits	4–5	6 oz. fruit juice;	apricots, bananas,

Food Group	Daily Servings (except as noted)	Serving Sizes	Examples
		1 medium fruit; ¼ cup dried fruit; ½ cup fresh, frozen, or canned fruit	dates, grapes, oranges, orange juice, grapefruit, grapefruit juice, mangoes, melons, peaches, pineapples, prunes, raisins, strawberries, tangerines
Low-fat or Fat free Dairy Foods	2–3	8 oz. milk; 1 cup yogurt; 1½ oz. cheese	fat free (skim) or low-fat (1%) milk, fat free or low-fat buttermilk, fat free or low-fat regular or frozen yogurt, fat free or low-fat cheese
Meat, Poultry, and Fish	2 or less	3 oz. cooked meats, poultry, or fish	lean only (trim away visible fats); broil, roast, or boil instead of frying; remove skin from poultry
Nuts, Seeds and Dry Beans	4–5 per week	⅓ cup or 1½ oz. nuts; 2 tbsp. seeds or ½ oz. seeds; ½ cup cooked dry beans	almonds, filberts mixed nuts, peanuts, walnuts, sunflower seeds, kidney beans, lentils, peas
Fats & Oils	2–3	1 tsp. soft margarine; 1 tbsp. low-fat mayonnaise; 2 tbsp. light salad dressing 1 tsp. vegetable oil	soft margarine, low-fat mayonnaise, light salad dressing, vegetable oil (such as olive, corn, canola, or safflower)
Sweets	5 per week	1 tbsp. sugar; 1 tbsp. jelly or jam; ½ oz. jelly beans	maple syrup, sugar, jelly, jam, fruit flavored gelatin, jelly beans, hard candy, fruit punch

National Cancer Institute Dietary Guidelines[4]

The National Cancer Institute recommends the following:

- Reduce intake of dietary fat to 30 percent of total calories or less.
- Increase fiber to 20 to 30 g per day with upper limits of 35 g
- Include a variety of fruits and vegetables in the daily diet.
- Avoid obesity.
- Consume alcoholic beverages in moderation, if at all.
- Minimize consumption of salt-cured, salt-pickled, and smoked foods.

American Institute for Cancer Research[5]

- Choose a diet rich in a variety of plant-based foods.
- Eat plenty of vegetables and fruit.
- Maintain a healthy weight and be physically active.
- Drink alcohol only in moderation, if at all.
- Select foods low in fat and salt.
- Prepare and store food safely.

And always remember . . . do not use tobacco in any form.

Source: Reprinted with permission from the American Institute for Cancer Research.

American Heart Association[6]

The American Heart Association recommends the following:

- Total fat intake should be less than 30 percent of calories.
- Saturated fatty acid intake should be 8 to 10 percent of calories.
- Polyunsaturated fatty acid intake should be up to 10 percent of calories.
- Monounsaturated fatty acids make up the rest of total fat intake, about 10 to 15 percent of total calories.
- Cholesterol intake should be less than 300 mg per day.
- Sodium intake should be no more than 2,400 mg (2.4 g) per day.

Source: Reproduced with permission. © The American Heart Association Diet, An Eating Plan for Healthy Americans: 51-2000, 1991–1996. Copyright American Heart Association.

American Heart Association[7]

The Association also recommends the following:

- Eat up to 6 ounces per day of (cooked) lean meat, fish, and skinless poultry.
- Try main dishes featuring pasta, rice, beans, and/or vegetables. Or create low-meat dishes by mixing these foods with small amounts of lean meat, poultry, or fish.
- The approximate 5- to 8-teaspoon servings of fats and oils per day may be used for cooking and baking, and in salad dressings and spreads.
- Use cooking methods that require little or no fat—boil, broil, bake, roast, poach, steam, sauté, stirfry or microwave.
- Trim off the fat you can see before cooking the meat and poultry. Drain off all fat after browning. Chill soups and stews after cooking so you can remove the hardened fat from the top.
- The three or four egg yolks per week included in your eating plan may be used alone or in cooking and baking (including store-bought products).
- Limit your use of organ meats such as liver, brains, chitterlings, kidney, heart, gizzard, sweetbreads, and pork maws.
- Choose skim or 1 percent fat milk and nonfat or low-fat yogurt and cheeses.

To round out the rest of your eating plan:

- Eat five or more servings of fruits or vegetables per day.
- Eat six or more servings of breads, cereals, or grains per day.

Source: Reproduced with permission. © The American Heart Association Diet, An Eating Plan for Healthy Americans, 1991–1996. Copyright American Heart Association.

American Cancer Society[8]

The following guidelines on diet, nutrition, and cancer prevention are provided by the American Cancer Society:

- Choose most of the foods you eat from plant sources.
- Eat five or more servings of fruits and vegetables each day.
- Eat other foods from plant sources, such as breads, cereals, grain products, rice, pasta, or beans several times each day.
- Limit your intake of high-fat foods, particularly from animal sources.
- Choose foods low in fat.
- Limit consumption of meats, especially high-fat meats.
- Be physically active: Achieve and maintain a healthy weight.
- Be at least moderately active for 30 minutes or more on most days of the week.
- Stay within your healthy weight range.
- Limit consumption of alcohol beverages, if you drink at all.

Source: Reprinted with permission from the American Cancer Society, Inc.

U.S. Department of Agriculture and U.S. Department of Health and Human Services.[9]

For a diet with plenty of grain products, vegetables, and fruits, eat daily: 6–11 servings of grain products (breads, cereals, pasta, and rice)

- Eat products made from a variety of whole grains, such as wheat, rice, oats, corn, and barley.
- Eat several servings of the whole-grain breads and cereals daily.
- Prepare and serve grain products with little or no fats and sugars.

3–5 servings of various vegetables and vegetable juices

- Choose dark-green leafy and deep-yellow vegetables often.
- Eat dry beans, peas, and lentils often.
- Eat starchy vegetables, such as potatoes and corn.
- Prepare and serve vegetables with little or no fats.

2–4 servings of various fruits and fruit juices

- Choose citrus fruits or juices, melons, or berries regularly.
- Eat fruits as desserts or snacks.
- Drink fruit juices.
- Prepare and serve fruits with little or no added sugars.

What Counts as a Serving?

Grain Products Group (bread, cereal, rice, and pasta)

- 1 slice of bread
- 1 ounce of ready-to-eat cereal
- ½ cup of cooked cereal, rice, or pasta

Vegetable Group

- 1 cup of leafy vegetables
- ½ cup of other vegetables—cooked or chopped raw
- ¾ cup of vegetable juice

Fruit Group

- 1 medium apple, banana, orange
- ½ cup of chopped, cooked, or canned fruit
- ¾ cup of fruit juice

Milk Group (milk, yogurt, and cheese)

- 1 cup of milk or yogurt
- 1½ ounces of natural cheese
- 2 ounces of processed cheese

Meats and Beans Group (meat, poultry, fish, dry beans, eggs, and nuts)

- 2–3 ounces of cooked lean meat, poultry, or fish
- ½ cup of dry beans or one egg counts as 1 ounce of meat. Two tablespoons of peanut butter or ⅓ cup of nuts count as 1 ounce of meat.

Source: U.S. Department of Agriculture and U.S. Department of Health and Human Services

American Heart Association[10]

Cholesterol Levels (Mg/dl)	Desirable (Low Risk)	Borderline-High Risk	High Risk
Total Cholesterol	less than 200	200–239	240 or higher
LDL (bad) Cholesterol	less than 130	130–159	160 or higher
HDL (good)	35 or higher	less than 35	less than 35

Source: Reproduced with permission. Copyright American Heart Association.

There appears to be a higher risk of coronary heart disease for women than for men with low HDL levels.[11] Forty percent of Americans have blood cholesterol levels greater than 200 mg per deciliter (dl), which doubles their risk for coronary heart disease compared to those with much lower cholesterol levels.[12]

Protein

Total protein intake should not be more than 15 percent of the total calories consumed. The RDA for a woman over age 25 is 0.75 g per kl of body weight per day. Depending on a woman's weight, protein intake should be approximately 30 to 70 g per day. This daily protein requirement can be satisfied by eating two eggs or 4 ounces of meat or chicken and a glass of milk.[13] One gram of protein is equal to 4 calories. High protein diets have been associated with increased loss of calcium in the urine, which can be detrimental to bone density. Animal protein sources are generally high in fats, which have been associated with heart disease, cancer, and weight gain.[14, 15]

Amino Acids

Twenty-two amino acids are known to be the building blocks of human protein. Nine of these cannot be synthesized by the body, and therefore must be assimilated from the diet; these are known as essential amino acids. The other thirteen are called nonessential amino acids since the body can manufacture them from other compounds. The intake of essential amino acids needs to be balanced or protein synthesis will be hampered.

Protein can be termed complete or incomplete. Complete protein contains eight of the nine essential amino acids. The ninth amino acid, histidine, is thought to be essential for infants and children, but probably not for adults. Incomplete protein lacks essential amino acids, therefore requiring other food sources to complete it. Complete protein foods are seafood, poultry, meat, eggs, cheese, and milk. Incomplete protein foods include grains, legumes, and other vegetables.

It is beyond the scope of this book to explore the research on amino acids. However, they are ingredients in many of the nutritional supplements on the market. As with vitamins and minerals, there are claims that we get all of our amino acid nutrients from an average diet and claims to the contrary.

Listed below are the amino acids:

Essential	**Nonessential**
Histidine	Alanine
Isoleucine	Arginine
Leucine	Asparagine
Lysine	Aspartic acid
Methionine	Cysteine
Phenylalanine	Cystine
Threonine	Glutamic acid
Tryptophan	Glutamine
Valine	Glycine
	Ornithine
	Proline
	Serine
	Tyrosine

Carbohydrates

Carbohydrates are the body's main source of calories or energy. They are generally classified as sugars or complex carbohydrates (starches).

Sugars

Sugars are simple carbohydrates that offer no vitamins or minerals. One gram of sucrose is equal to four calories. Common sugars are either monosaccharides or disaccharides (i.e., they are made up of one basic sugar unit or two units linked together). The monosaccharides are glucose (dextrose), fructose, and galactose. Disaccharides are combinations of these in double units.

Sucrose, from sugar beets and sugar cane, is plain table sugar. It is a disaccharide composed of the monosaccharides fructose and glucose. Both of these are found in fruits and honey. Fructose is also made commercially from cornstarch. Other disaccharides are lactose and maltose. Lactose is milk sugar. Maltose is malt sugar, used in the fermentation of beer, a product of breadmaking, and found in legumes.

The average person in the United States consumes about 125 pounds of sugar per year. This is equivalent to approximately 18 percent of total calories consumed. Consuming the average of two pounds of sugar per week represents 3,600 calories, the equivalent of almost one pound of fat. Reducing sugars is a helpful way to reduce weight gain.[16,17] Also, too much sugar can lead to tooth decay and can also predispose postmenopausal women to vaginitis by raising the vaginal pH, inviting infection.[18]

How do you reduce sugar in your diet? Here are some simple tips you may find helpful:

- Read ingredient labels. Identify all the added sugars in a product. Select items lower in added sugars when possible.
- Buy fresh fruits or fruits packed in water, juice, or light syrup rather than those in heavy syrup.
- Buy fewer foods that are high in sugars such as soft drinks, fruit-flavored punches and ades, and sweet desserts. Be aware that some low-fat desserts may be high in sugars.
- Reach for fresh fruit instead of something sweetened with additional sugars for dessert or a snack.
- Add less sugar to food—coffee, tea, cereal, or fruit. Get used to using half as much, then see if you can cut back even more.

Complex Carbohydrates

Complex carbohydrates (starches and dietary fiber) are long strands of simple sugars. Many health agencies recommend that half the calories consumed be from carbohydrates. Carbohydrates have been linked to a reduction in the risks of colon cancer and heart disease. They are found in grains, peas, beans, fruits, potatoes, and vegetables. One gram of carbohydrate is equal to four calories.

Starches

Starches, such as potatoes and pastas, are good food sources for energy, maintaining weight, and preventing obesity. Starches by themselves are not high in calories; it is all the high-calorie stuff people put on them that makes them fattening.[19]

Fiber

Fiber is the nondigestible parts of plants. It also consists of complex carbohydrates made up of long chains of simple sugars. But the sugars are linked together differently than they are in starch, and our digestive enzymes can't break them down. Diets high in fiber may help prevent digestive disorders, hemorrhoids, cancer of the colon and rectum, help with weight management, and lower serum cholesterol levels.[20] The National Cancer Institute recommends 20 to 30 g of fiber per day.

Fiber can be either soluble or insoluble. Soluble fiber is found in beans, fruits, oat bran, vegetables, and brown rice. It may help lower blood cholesterol levels. Insoluble fiber is found in whole grain products and again in fruits and vegetables. It helps provide bulk that is necessary for the formation of stools.

Diets high in fiber may inhibit the absorption of some minerals and vitamins. Women who eat high fiber diets may have an increased need for both calcium and magnesium.[21]

Fats

Fats are a necessary part of the diet. They are needed among other things for energy, for cell membrane structure, and to transport fat-soluble nutrients such as vitamins A, D, E, and K throughout the body. Most health agencies recommend that less than 30 percent of total calories come from fats and less than 10 percent from saturated fats. One gram of fat is equal to nine calories, so the above recommendation translates into 66 g of fat in a 2,000-calorie diet. The following are different types of fats:[22]

Triglycerides

A term that often comes up in the discussion of fat is triglycerides. They are fats made up of three fatty acids attached to a glycerol molecule. In the body, these are the major transport and storage form of fats. They are also the major form of fats in food. High levels of triglycerides have been associated with heart disease and diabetes.

Cholesterol

A fat-like substance, cholesterol is both manufactured by the body and consumed in the diet, mostly from animal sources. It is needed to make bile salts, hormones, and vitamin D. High cholesterol levels have been associated with increased risk of heart disease. Cholesterol is found in animal products, dairy products, fish, and shellfish.

Monounsaturated Fats

Primarily found in olive, canola, and peanut oil, monounsaturated fats may help to lower cholesterol levels, increase HDL and reduce LDL, reducing the risk of heart disease. High intakes of monounsaturated fats are negatively associated with breast cancer.[23, 24]

Polyunsaturated Fats

Poyunsaturated oils are mostly vegetable oils that are liquid at room temperature. Some are omega-6 oils such as soybean, safflower, corn, sunflower, sesame, and cottonseed. Also in this group are the omega-3 fish oils, which have been shown to lower blood cholesterol levels. (See Chapter 27.) It is been suggested that the balance of omega-3 and omega-6 in the diet may explain many of the international differences between the incidence of breast cancer around the world. A higher ratio of omega-3 to omega-6 appears to be more protective. It was even suggested that dietary intervention over a three-month period could positively influence breast cancer growth.[25] Another study, taking biopsies from women with abnormalities and metastatic breast cancer, compared the fatty acid profiles of breast tissue. N-3 fatty acids had a protective effect; N-6 and trans-fatty acids were associated with higher risk of breast cancer.[26]

Saturated Fats

Saturated fats are generally found in animal products and some vegetable oils. They are usually solid at room temperature. Saturated fats are known to raise the cholesterol levels in the blood, increasing the risk of heart disease. Saturated fats are found in meats, dairy products, some fatty fish, coconut oil, palm oil, palm kernel oil, whipped toppings, and nondairy coffee creamers. In a study where dietary patterns of fat consumption were studied, four patterns were investigated:

1. High total dietary lipids (high intake of mostly saturated animal lipids) resulted in high cancer rates and high coronary artery disease.
2. High total dietary lipids (low animal lipids) resulted in intermediate cancer and low coronary artery disease.
3. Moderate total dietary lipids (low to moderate animal lipids) resulted in intermediate cancer and low coronary artery disease.
4. Low total dietary lipids (low animal lipids) resulted in low cancer rates and low coronary artery disease.

The cancer rates were of the breast, prostate, and large bowel.[27]

Trans-Fatty Acids

In the United States, daily per capita animal fat consumption decreased from 104 g in 1909 to 97 g in 1972, while the consumption of vegetable fats increased from 21 to 59 g. Thus animal fats decreased from 83 to 62 percent as a proportion of our total fat intake.[28] This was over a period of time that authorities were diligently warning us about the dangers of animal fats predisposing to heart disease and cancer. But while heart disease and cancer rates were rising, the consumption of animal fats was falling. Something didn't make sense. That something may well be trans-fatty acids.

As early as the 1950s, researchers posed a concern over processed vegetable fats and their effect on health. A process called *hydrogenation* is used to transform unsaturated vegetable oils such as soybean oil into less saturated oils and fats. This accomplishes two things. It gives them a longer shelf life, with less tendency to become rancid. And it can convert oils into fats, that is, oils that are solid at room temperature. The latter can be used for margarine, spreads, and shortenings. Today partially hydrogenated vegetable shortenings have largely replaced lard, butter, and other animal fats in the U.S. baking industry. However, synthetic hydrogenation produces trans-fatty acids, chemically altered unsaturated fatty acids that have a different type of carbon-carbon double bond than is found in naturally occurring fats. According to estimates, the daily per capita intake of trans-fatty acids rose from 4.4 g in 1910 to 12.1 g in 1972.[29] A more recent figure indicates the average consumption is between 8 and 15 g.[30]

Unfortunately it has taken about 30 years for these concerns to be given serious attention, but recent literature has more and more studies critical of trans-fatty acids. These fats have been shown to raise LDL cholesterol and lower HDLs,[31] alter immune response, change cell membrane structure, and, perhaps most ominously alter some enzyme systems that metabolize carcinogens and drugs.[32] Indeed, some investigators have found associations between trans-fatty acids and increased risk of heart disease in women[33] as well as breast cancer.[34] A study of 698 European postmenopausal women with primary breast cancer had gluteal fat biopsies measured. Women with higher trans-fatty acids in their adipose tissue had a higher risk of breast cancer. This was thought to be due to a high dietary intake of trans-fatty acids and/or trans-fatty acids altering the metabolism of other fatty acids.[35]

Researchers at the Harvard School of Public Health take the relationship between trans-fatty acids and coronary artery disease very seriously. They believe that trans-fatty acids in partially hydrogenated oils are responsible for at least 30,000 premature deaths per year in the United States.[36] The same researchers have called for federal regulations to greatly reduce or eliminate the use of partially hydrogenated vegetable fat.[37] Until that happens, try to avoid them.

Try to eat monounsaturated fats in favor of other fats and limit the use of polyunsaturated fats, especially hydrogenated vegetable oils. Cookies, donuts, deep-fried foods, chips, imitation cheese, and pastries not made with butter or lard are full of trans-fatty acids from partially hydrogenated oils,[38] so are margarine and spreads, but, in general, the softer the item, the less hydrogenation. For example, liquid or tub margarine has less hydrogenation than stick margarine.[39] And finally, avoid olestra.

Olestra

Olestra was developed in 1968 in an attempt to find an efficient way to get extra calories into premature babies. That tack was abandoned when it was realized that olestra was nondigestible. Olestra looked like fat, felt like fat, and tasted like fat; but it had no calories since it wasn't digested or absorbed—What a great diet fat! However, even though it has been approved by the FDA for use of in the food industry, all olestra products must have warning labels about causing abdominal cramps and loose stools. Individuals have also commonly reported problems such as fecal urgency and flatulence. These problems are generally transient and range from mild to quite severe.[40] Besides causing gastrointestinal problems, olestra may also increase the risk of cancer, heart disease, and blindness by reducing carotenoid levels. Some epidemiologists have found it puzzling that the same government that is encouraging its citizens to eat more fruits and fresh vegetables for their carotenoids has approved a chemical that depletes them.[41] Study after study show that olestra inhibits the absorption of carotenoids and lycopene.[42, 43, 44]

Tips for Fat Reduction

From the technical to the practical, following are some smart methods of fat reduction in the diet:

- Eat more fruits, vegetables, and their juices. Most are naturally low in fat and high in vitamins and minerals.
- Choose low-fat or nonfat products at the supermarket. For example, pretzels, depending on the brand, have little to no fat as compared to regular potato chips or corn chips. Angel food cake would be a better choice than devil's food cake. When shopping for spreads, select soft-

tub margarine over regular stick margarine—the better choice if you are going to eat them at all. It is probably wiser to eat real butter and just make sure the total saturated fat in your diet does not exceed 10 percent.

- Use lean meats. Sounds great, but what does it mean and how do you select lean? When shopping, look at the type of cut; loin and round in the title is an indication that it is a leaner cut of meat. White meat poultry has less fat than dark meat poultry. Lean ham is a better choice than bacon or sausage. And how much meat should you eat? Typically no more than 5 to 7 ounces per day. As a guide, the recommended size of one serving (3 oz.) of cooked meat is about the size of a deck of cards.
- When heading down the dairy aisle, keep these things in mind. Skim milk or nonfat milk should be your choice. Whole milk contains 8 grams of fat per 8 ounce glass. Buttermilk made with skim milk is a low-fat alternative to whole milk. A good substitute for half-and-half or cream is evaporated skim milk.
- This same logic applies when selecting cheeses and other dairy products. If you are making lasagna, substitute low-fat ricotta for regular cheese. The flavor remains the same, but the calories and fat are substantially reduced. Nonfat or low-fat yogurts are far better for you than regular yogurts, yet provide the same amount of calcium.
- Rounding the corner and heading for the desserts, there is a large variety of nonfat and low-fat puddings and frozen sweets. Today's most popular brands are usually available in low-fat or nonfat varieties. Be sure to read the label. Look for the amount of fat the product contains. Low-fat or no-fat ice creams, yogurts, ices, and puddings top the list. Many of these low- and no-fat varieties taste as good as the traditional products. Remember, even if the product is low in fat, it still contains calories, so portion is still an important consideration.
- Almost every product in the supermarket today has a low-fat or no-fat counterpart. Breads and pastas follow suit. Add these considerations to your shopping list: Bagels are

better than doughnuts, and English muffins contain less fat than croissants. Here again, the topping or spread you choose can easily add calories and fat to your meal.

- To help cut the total fat in cooking, limit the amount to 5 to 8 teaspoons per day. Bake, broil, boil, steam, poach, or microwave foods instead of frying, and substitute high-fat ingredients with low-fat alternatives. In place of regular oil, use a nonstick cooking spray. Egg whites or egg substitutes are a good no-cholesterol substitute for whole eggs. As a general guide, use two egg whites for each whole egg, or use egg substitutes.
- Supermarket shopping can be overwhelming because there are so many choices. To relieve this job, during each trip to the store pick one aisle and review the labels for their contents. Try to avoid foods that are high in fats and sodium. Avoid foods with hydrogenated fats or oils (this is extremely hard to find on the label). And try to find foods that contain more "food" than chemicals, preservatives, and words that you do not understand. Keep a list of the good-for-you items, and, next trip, pick a new aisle.

Sodium

As the body ages, kidney function slows down, and the body is less able to rid itself of excess sodium. Too much sodium in the diet may increase the risk of high blood pressure, kidney failure, and heart disease. Many health agencies recommend that people eat less than 3 g of sodium per day. The average person in the United States consumes about 6 to 8 g of sodium per day. Our bodies only require 0.5 g of salt or 0.2 g of sodium per day. Generally 30 percent of salt intake comes from the use of salt at the table and in food preparation, and 70 percent is derived from that naturally present in foods and from commercial processing of foods. Other sources of sodium include:[45,46]

- Baking soda
- Baking powder
- Monosodium glutamate
- Sodium caseinate
- Sodium saccharin
- Sodium benzoate
- Disodium phosphate
- Sodium nitrate

- Sodium citrate
- Some antacids
- Sodium hydroxide
- Sodium sulfite
- Some sleeping aids
- Sodium alginate
- Sodium propionate

Reducing sodium intake is one of the first reasonable approaches in managing blood pressure in hypertensive women.[47] To help you reduce sodium in your diet, try the following suggestions.

- Read labels on processed foods to identify the sodium content of a serving. Select fresh or plain frozen vegetables and meats instead of those canned with salt. Look for low-sodium, or no-salt-added versions of such foods as: canned vegetables, vegetable juices, dried soup mixes, bouillon condiments (catsup, soy sauce), snack foods (chips, nuts, pretzels), crackers, bakery products, canned soups, and processed meats.
- Cook rice, pasta, and hot cereals without salt or using less salt than the package calls for (try ⅛ teaspoon salt for two servings). Adjust your recipes, gradually cutting down on the amount of salt. Experiment with the flavors of lemon or lime juice, herbs, and spices as seasonings for vegetables and meats instead of salt.
- Leave the salt shaker off the table.

Water

A woman's body is composed of about 60 percent water. Water helps carry nutrients, hormones, and oxygen throughout the body. It also is responsible for flushing out waste products. According to recommendations, a woman should drink six 8-ounce glasses of water per day.[48] To help you drink more water, try the following tips:

- Choose juice, milk, or sparkling water for a snack or to complement a meal. Take a water break instead of a coffee break.

- When working at your desk, keep a container or glass of water handy to sip on throughout the day.
- Keep a supply of bottled water handy on trips or outings.

Alcohol

The jury is still out on the effects of alcohol. Some say that longevity is increased in moderate drinkers. Alcohol does have an overall positive effect of raising HDL3 (a subfraction of HDL), but it is disputed whether this provides any protection against coronary heart disease. It also has been shown to increase blood pressure and impair glucose tolerance. Alcohol depletes vitamin A, thiamin, riboflavin, biotin, choline, B6, folic acid, niacin, calcium, and magnesium.[49] Some of the effects of drinking alcohol are insomnia, liver damage, depression, increased susceptibility to infection, inhibition of the immune system, and increased risk of high blood pressure and cancer. Alcohol is considered a risk factor for breast cancer. It also promotes hot flashes during the climacterium.[50, 51]

If you are going to drink, drink in moderation. What is moderation? Moderation is defined as no more than one drink per day for women and no more than two drinks per day for men.

The following count as one drink:

- 12 ounces of regular beer (150 calories)
- 5 ounces of wine (100 calories)
- 1.5 ounces of 80-proof distilled spirits (100 calories)

Caffeine

Caffeine and its relationship to health has been explored throughout the years. Some studies have shown that caffeine constricts the blood vessels, elevates body temperature, causes high blood pressure, and can trigger hot flashes. Caffeine depletes vitamin C, calcium, zinc, potassium, and the B vitamins.[52] The tannins in coffee or tea reduce the absorption of many minerals, especially iron. It was suggested that less than two cups of coffee a day will not have any negative health risks.[53] Most people can enjoy caffeine-containing beverages. For most healthy women, moderate caffeine intake of 200 to 300 mg a day (the amount in two cups of coffee) should pose no problems. If you are caffeine sensitive and have been advised by your physician to restrict the amount of caffeine you consume, here are some ideas to help you decaffeinate your intake:

- Cut back gradually, since sudden withdrawal can cause headaches and drowsiness, especially if you are used to ingesting a lot of caffeine.
- Read labels on medicines since caffeine is an ingredient in more than 1,000 over-the-counter drugs.
- Read labels on soft drinks. Caffeine is also an ingredient in more than 75 percent of the soft drinks consumed.
- Try decaffeinated beverages, or mix regular with some decaffeinated coffee.

The tea that is consumed in China and Japan has properties equivalent to vitamin E supplements. Green and black tea are antioxidants. Black tea is a fermented product of green tea.[54] Although the studies are inconclusive, there is evidence of a protective effect of tea consumption against cancer.[55]

Like any other changes in behavior or lifestyle we make, how we select foods and the amount we eat require willpower and adjustments. This chapter clearly provides well-researched information and evidence as to what's good for you and your overall health. You are the one walking down the aisles of the supermarket and making the selections. When it is time for meal preparation, you decide what is best for you and your family.

29

The Female Heart

BREAST CANCER AND osteoporosis have received top billing as women's health issues because they are "women's diseases." But cardiovascular disease, a supposedly male problem, is *the* major cause of death in women over 50 years old. One of every three women will die of heart disease. In 1993 over a half million women in the United States died from heart disease, 250,000 died from all forms of cancer (including 43,600 women with breast cancer[1]), and fewer than 2 percent of women older than 65 died from osteoporosis-related hip fractures.[2] A woman is twice as likely to die in the two weeks following a heart attack than is a man. One in seven women between the ages of 45 and 64 has some form of heart disease. This rate increases to one in three after the age of 65.[3] Coronary heart disease is 1.9 times as likely to occur in inactive people than in people who exercise. More than half the people living in the United States have blood cholesterol levels greater than 200 mg per dl, which puts them at risk for coronary heart disease. Most studies on exercise and heart disease have been conducted on young and middle-aged men. The studies on women and girls are limited, and results of the studies are inconclusive.[4]

The Heart

The normal heart is a muscle that acts as a pump, moving about 2,000 gallons of blood a day. The heart beats, filling and contracting, about 100,000 times a day. The heart consists of four chambers: The top two are called *atria*, and the bottom two are called *ventricles*. Blood is pumped through them in an organized and systematic fashion. Four valves control the one-way directional flow of blood. The right side of the heart is a relatively low-pressure system, pumping blood from the body to the lungs; and the left side is a high-pressure system, pumping blood from the lungs to the body.

First, the right atrium fills with blood, which has traveled throughout the body and has returned to the heart via the veins. This blood has a high saturation of carbon dioxide and a low saturation of oxygen. When the atria contract, blood flows into the right ventricle. Next, the ventricles contract, which pushes the blood into the pulmonary artery and on to the lungs. While in the lungs, the carbon dioxide in the blood diffuses into the *alveoli* (small, bubble-like sacs in the lungs) and is expelled. At the same time, in the other direction, oxygen diffuses across the alveolar membranes and is picked up by hemoglobin in the blood. Thus replenished, oxygenated blood then flows into the left atrium, through the mitral valve, and then into the left ventricle. With another ventricular contraction, the oxygenated blood is pushed through the *aorta*, the body's major artery, and is distributed throughout the entire circulatory system.

The circulatory system is a network of elastic tubing that takes oxygen and nutrients to all parts of the body. This system also picks up the body's waste products and delivers them to the liver, lungs, and kidneys where they are filtered, excreted, exchanged, or metabolized.

Women should be particularly aware of a common heart condition of young people called *mitral valve prolapse* (MVP), which is estimated to occur in about 4 to 15 percent of the general population[5], but is more common in women and is often an inherited trait.[6] Prolapse refers to a bulging of the valve leaflets backward into the left atrium during ventricular contraction. It may or may not be associated with *mitral regurgitation* (backflow of blood from the left ventricle into the left atrium during ventricular contraction). The condition exists in a wide spectrum of severity, from just an interesting medical finding to something that will cause heart failure. It may or may not be associated with symptoms of palpitation, fatigue, and chest pain. Furthermore, the severity of the condition may not correlate with the degree of prolapse or regurgitation. Women with reason to believe they have heart symptoms of prolapse should be examined by a cardiologist and if warranted have an echocardiogram done to determine the presence and degree of regurgitation. Women with no murmur or evidence of regurgitation can be reassured of their benign condition.[7] For the remaining patients, treatment and follow-up depend on the severity of the situation. Most experts agree that women with evidence of regurgitation should receive prophylactic antibiotics prior to teeth cleaning, dental work, and surgery to prevent bacterial infection of the heart valve (endocarditis).

Diet and the Heart

Diet has been shown to be a major player in the development of heart disease, and reduction of fat and salt intake is urged. As is widely known, excess salt consumption is one of the common contributors to high blood pressure, which in turn contributes to heart disease and stroke. Approximately half the women over age 55 have high blood pressure. Black women have a death rate from high blood pressure almost five times that of white women.[8] Blood pressure is written as a fraction. The top number is the systolic and the bottom number is the diastolic. Optimal blood pressure would be less than 120/80, normal is 120–129/85, high normal is 130–139/85–90, and high is 140/90 and above. A woman routinely should have her blood pressure checked every 2½ years. High blood pressure usually causes no symptoms until it causes some catastrophic event such as stroke or heart attack, so don't wait until you "feel like your blood pressure is up" to be checked.

The American Heart Association[9]

Blood Pressure (mm Hg)	Optimal	Normal	High Normal	Hypertension
Systolic (top number)	less than 120	less than 130	130–139	140 or higher
Diastolic (bottom number)	less than 80	less than 85	85–90	90 or higher

Source: Reproduced with permission. American Heart Association.

More fascinating, however, is the recent concern over trans-fatty acids, commonly found in partially hydrogenated vegetable fats and oils. It turns out that the rise in heart disease in America more closely follows the increase in use of these oils than it does the consumption of animal fats, which has actually declined since 1900.[10] (For more on trans-fatty acids and for the American Heart Association Dietary Guidelines, see Chapter 28.)

Homocysteine is an amino acid that has been in the forefront lately in a whole host of pathological conditions. Many recent studies have indicated that elevated plasma levels of homocysteine are associated with increased risk of coronary atherosclerosis, cerebrovascular disease, peripheral vascular disease, and thrombosis. In fact, evidence shows that homocysteine is a direct causal factor for these problems. High levels of homocysteine may be the result of a genetic trait, lifestyle, or nutritional problem. Young women with elevated plasma homocysteine and low plasma folate are at increased risk for myocardial infarction.[11] Three vitamins—B_{12}, B_6, and folate—are needed to appropriately metabolize homocysteine, and not surprisingly intakes of folate, B_6, and B_{12} are inversely associated with plasma homocysteine levels.[12] In a study of approximately 500 people, the subjects with the lowest B_{12} and folate values had significantly higher homocysteine concentrations than the people with higher vitamin levels.[13] In another study, people taking multivitamins containing, among other vitamins, only 200 to 400 mcg of folic acid had significantly lower plasma homocysteine levels (–22 percent) than subjects not taking multivitamins.[14]

Levels of homocysteine can be reduced with pharmacologic doses of folic acid, B_6, and B_{12}.[15, 16, 17] One to 5 mg of folate along with B vitamins can normalize plasma homocysteine levels. Antioxidants E and C can also be used to reduce homocysteine-related oxidative stress.[18]

Chlamydia Pneumonia Infection

People usually don't think of arteriosclerosis as an infectious disease, but recently chlamydia pneumonia infection has been associated with atherosclerosis and increased risk of stroke. It is suspected that a low-grade, chronic infection of the lining of the arteries causes an inflammation that makes the vessel walls more susceptible to the development of atherosclerotic plaque. This germ is found in both gum disease and bronchitis. In fact, gum diseases may be associated with doubling the risk of stroke. So go to the dentist and have regular checkups. The infection is treatable, and you may reduce your cardiovascular risk.[19, 20]

Studies support supplementing with vitamin E. (See Chapter 7.) Studies also support supplementing with CoQ_{10}. (See Chapter 9.)

Heart Care

Take care of your heart:

- Do not smoke!
- Exercise and be active.
- ERT/HRT is effective in reducing the risk of cardiovascular disease. However, the protective effects disappear three years after stopping.[21]
- Avoid eating trans-fatty acids and olestra.
- Red wine with meals may have a cardio-protective effect.
- Take a vitamin and mineral supplement with B_6, B_{12}, folic acid, niacin, E, C, CoQ_{10}, calcium, and magnesium.
- Reduce meat consumption. Replace with fish and soy products.
- Consume lots of fruits and vegetables.

Warning

Women generally have fewer and less severe symptoms of heart attack than do men. Take unusual chest, stomach, or abdominal pain seriously. Other symptoms are nausea, dizziness, shortness of breath or difficulty in breathing, unexplained anxiety, weakness, fatigue, palpitations, cold sweats, or paleness. It is imperative to get help as soon as possible. Damage to the heart and brain can be reduced if treated in the first few hours. One reason women do poorly with heart attacks is that treatment is often delayed because either they or their doctors do not seriously consider the possibility of a heart attack. So be defensively suspicious!

30

Herbs

For centuries, plants have been used around the world for medicinal purposes. Generally, in the United States, plants have been replaced by synthetic products. However, there seems to be a reawakening of interest in the use of plants for health and medicinal purposes. This is demonstrated by the number of fast-growing herbal companies that have opened their doors in the past few years.

There is little room to doubt that many plants have medicinal value. Yet there are problems inherent in their administration and use. To begin with, determining dosage is difficult. Controlling quality in a plant is extremely difficult. The concentration or potency of the constituents in each plant is determined by the soil, location, climate, season, and other uncontrollable factors. Second there often exist in the plant nonbeneficial or even harmful substances that ideally should be avoided. Third, the optimal durations of herbal therapies are unknown. Fourth, little information is available on the short- and long-term side-effects of various herbs. And last, most of the information available on herbal therapy is based on anecdotal testimonies and folklore, not rigorous scientific research. Few scientific studies have been done, most of the them animal-based.

These are not problems limited to "radical" herbal medicine. Up until a few years ago, many of these previous statements could have been made (and were) about one of the most widely used heart drugs in the world—digitalis, an extract of foxglove. Debate continued for years over the advantages of various extracted components versus pills made from the whole leaf. One of the major problems with both treatment and research was the inability to standardize dosage, since the potency of the product varied greatly according to source, growing conditions of the foxglove, etc. Two lessons learned from the "herbal research" on digitalis and heart disease were that dosage standardization is difficult and that too much of a wonderful thing can be poisonous.

The present discussion will be limited to garlic, onions, some plants producing estrogenic effects, and a few herbs most commonly used for female problems. Garlic is actually recognized by the Japanese FDA as a treatment for hypertension. Both garlic and onions have been researched for their value in reducing blood cholesterol and cancer risk. Soybeans have been researched for their value in inhibiting the growth of certain cancers and their role in lowering the risk of breast cancer. Still other plants produce chemical compounds that exhibit estrogenic activity in both humans and animals; these chemicals are called *phytoestrogens* (i.e., plant estrogens.) This group of plants includes soybeans, yams, apple, barley, carrot, winter cherry, coffee, green beans, oats, parsley, peas, pomegranate, potato, red beans, rape, rice, rye, sesame, wheat, yeast, ginseng, licorice, fennel, unicorn root, false unicorn root, alfalfa, red clover, dong quai, sage, and black cohosh.[1, 2] In addition, phytoestrogens have been identified in beer (containing hops) and bourbon (made from corn).[3]

Garlic and Onion

In a review of the genus *Allium*, both garlic and onion were shown to be effective inhibitors of platelet aggregation (essential for clotting) in human blood. They were also shown to prevent increases of plasma fibrinogen and reductions in blood coagulation time and fibrinolytic activity. In plain English, this means that garlic and onion may help lower the risk of blood clots and thereby reduce the risk of strokes. Onion and garlic have also been shown to reduce serum cholesterol and triglycerides.[4] In Germany, Kwai (a Chinese garlic) is licenced as a drug for the treatment of atherosclerosis; in the United States, it is considered a dietary supplement.[5] People who eat as little as 10 g (1/3 oz.) per week of garlic and 200 g (6 to 7 oz.) per week of onion were better protected than people who abstain. However, those who eat 50 g (almost 2 oz.) per week of garlic and 600 g (20 oz.) per week of onion show even greater benefits.[6] In a recent review of placebo-controlled, randomized studies, it was ascertained that high-cholesterol patients could reduce their cholesterol levels by an average of 9 percent by eating as little as one-half to one clove (not bulb) of garlic daily.[7]

In a double-blind, placebo-controlled study, subjects who took 800 mg of garlic powder per day over a four-week period had significant beneficial changes in their blood: inhibited blood clot development, increased capillary circulation, and decreased blood sugar values. These blood changes possibly could have an effect on reducing the risk of heart disease and helping patients with diabetes.[8]

Garlic consumption was shown to be strongly associated with low risk of colon cancer in a 1994 study, with a 35 percent reduction of risk among garlic eaters. This was a more striking association than was found with any other fruits, vegetables, or dietary fiber studied in a group of more than 40,000 women.[9] Epidemiological studies in China have shown that the dietary intake of garlic is inversely related to the incidence of gastric cancer.[10]

Fresh garlic also has been shown to be effective as an antibacterial agent against both Gram-positive and Gram-negative organisms, even against strains of some organisms that have become resistant to common antibiotics. The compound allicin is the active antibacterial agent in garlic, and its use or that of synthetic analogues as antibacterial agents is worth further exploration.[11]

Phytoestrogens

Phytoestrogens were first studied in the 1920s. To date approximately 300 different plants are known to produce these compounds, which are about 1/400th as potent as estradiol in the human body.[12] Phytoestrogens are not actually estrogens, but they can bind to estrogen receptors and elicit a similar response.[13] The three main groups of phytoestrogens are lignans, coumestans, and isoflavones. Tamoxifen, a drug widely used to treat breast cancer, has a structure similar to some phytoestrogens.[14] It also has been used as a preventative drug for women who are at high risk for breast cancer. In a six-year study, tamoxifen cut women's risk of breast cancer in half and lowered the risk of fractures. However, the drug doubles the risk of endometrial cancer and increases risk of blood clots in the lungs and deep veins.[15]

Estrogen receptors are very complex and not well understood. It is thought that the phytoestrogenic agents work in the following manner: There are a limited number of estrogen receptors in the body. They can be occupied by either estrogen or phytoestrogen or can be vacant. If the majority are bound by estrogen, the estrogenic activity is high. If the majority are vacant, the estrogenic activity is low. Introduction of phytoestrogens moderates this situation. In low estrogen states, phytoestrogens will increase estrogenic activity by binding to empty sites. In high estrogen states, they will reduce estrogenic activity by displacing some of the estrogen molecules with less potent substitutes. Michael Murray and Joseph Pizzorno, the authors of *Encyclopedia of Natural Medicine*, add that, as opposed to estrogen, phytoestrogens have not been associated with an increased risk of cancer.[16]

In the past three years, research in this area has increased tremendously. Study after study show the beneficial effects of phytoestrogens on reducing osteoporosis, heart disease, cholesterol, hormone independent cancers, and colon cancer.[17, 18, 19, 20]

Soybeans, clover and alfalfa sprouts, and oil seeds (such as flaxseed) are the most significant dietary sources of isoflavones, coumestans, and lignans.[21] Isoflavones, particularly genistein and daidzein are found in soy and garbanzo beans. These are mostly found in products like tempeh, soy, miso, and tofu. Coumestans have a light steroid activity. High concentrations are found in red clover, sunflower seeds, and bean sprouts. Lignans, a constituent of the cell wall of plants, are found in seed oils, mostly flaxseed.

Soybeans are probably the most thoroughly researched of the phytoestrogen-producing plants. Soybeans also contain a few different anticarcinogens and growth inhibitors. Two of these agents, genistein and daidzein, have been shown to inhibit or prevent the development of experimentally induced colon, lung, liver, oral, and esophageal cancers in animals.[22] A recent study conducted on Japanese men and women who ate a traditional Japanese diet concluded that the low incidence of breast and prostate cancer among the Japanese may be linked to their high intake of soybeans.[23] A traditional Japanese diet derives between 20 and 60 percent of the protein from soybeans. The Japanese eat 36.1 g of tofu, 15.3 g of miso, 8 g of tofu products, and 7 g of other soy products daily. Western Europeans (Americans) only eat a few mg of soy products per day.[24]

Phytochemicals are derived from plants, and xenoestrogens are derived from industrial, agricultural, or other environmental sources. Much research is needed to clarify the difference between plant-based estrogens and industrial xenoestrogens. However, the phytochemicals' effects are relatively short-lived, with positive effects, whereas the xenoestrogens' effects are longer acting, and some are suspected to be cancer causing.[25] Xenoestrogens disrupt normal endrocrine functions, leading to reproductive failure and cancer of estrogen-sensitive tissues. Phytoestrogens may block binding of xenoestrogens to estrogen receptors, negating the harmful effects; however, since they are so short-lived, they may not be of practical benefit.[26]

Some interesting effects from phytoestrogens have been recorded. According to Hopkins et al., uterine bleeding in a postmenopausal woman was caused by the use of a Chinese ginseng face cream; the phytoestrogens absorbed through her skin had been enough to influence her uterine lining.[27] Another study showed that premenopausal women consuming soy protein isolate daily for six months had stimulatory effect on their breasts.[28] In animals, sterility problems have been attributed to the consumption of phytoestrogens. Sterility has been reported in Australian sheep grazing on subterranean clover, a phytoestrogen-producing plant.[29] Infertility and liver disease are common problems seen in captive cheetahs fed diets high in soy protein. Researchers concluded that soy isoflavones in the diet are likely responsible.[30] A contraceptive effect was also noted in a study on rabbits and rats fed castor plant (*Ricinus communis* var. *minor*) seeds.[31] These results were also found in a study on rats given injections of extracts of winter cherry fruit, a traditional contraceptive recommended by Iranian herbalists. The rats had a 96 percent reduction of pups and their progesterone levels decreased by 44 percent. When the treatments stopped the pregnancy rate increased to normal levels.[32]

There is enough evidence to warrant soy protein supplements following primary surgery for early breast cancer. It is a safe diet and allows a woman to participate in her treatment plan.[33]

Until recently yams were a major source of medicinal estrogen products. They were eventually replaced with synthetic and animal estrogens. Premarin, a conjugated estrogen, is derived from *pre*gnant *mare*'s ur*ine*, an abundant and inexpensive source of estrogen.[34]

Herbs Commomly Used for Female Disorders

Recently there has been an explosion of availability of preformulated vitamin, mineral, and herbal remedies available from retail stores, mail-order houses, and multilevel marketing businesses. A close reading of the labels will often find one or more of the following herbs in the preparation. The brief descriptions will provide the rationale for their inclusion in the mixture. *Warning*: All contraindications that apply to estrogen use also apply to the use of herbs with phytoestrogens. (See Chapter 25.) Not enough data are available at this time to recommend the use of these herbs without warning.

Phytoestrogen Herbs

Dong Quai

This common Chinese root has been used medicinally for more than 2,000 years. It regulates the menstrual cycle, reduces menstrual pain, reduces abdominal pain, and increases vaginal lubrication. The side effects of dong quai are mild and rare. Contraindications are diarrhea, hemorrhagic disease, hypermenorrhea, first three months of pregnancy, spontaneous abortion, and use during flu or cold.[35] Dong quai used alone does not produce estrogen-like responses in endometrial thickness or vaginal maturation. It was no more helpful than a placebo in relieving menopausal problems.[36]

Ginseng

There are three different types of ginseng: Siberian, American, and Panax. Panax is the most widely used. The roots seem to increase activity of the adrenal glands and are touted to increase sexual endurance. Estrogen-like effects were seen in the vaginal lining of postmenopausal women taking Panax ginseng for a two-week period.[37] A study of 503 patients who were given either a multivitamin with ginseng or the multivitamin alone for a 12-week period reported on a follow-up questionnaire that the multivitamin with ginseng was more effective in improving the quality of life.[38] Taking echinacea and ginseng (Panax) together was shown to enhance natural killer cell activity functions in both normal patients and those with depressed cellular immunity.[39] *Warning*: Ginseng can raise blood pressure.

Sage

This herb has been used to regulate menstrual flow and relieve hot flashes.

Black Cohosh

The roots and rhizomes of black cohosh supposedly help cramps associated with menstruation and relieve hot flashes and excessive bleeding. The herb has been administered during childbirth to reduce pain and stimulate uterine contractions. *Warning*: Large doses can cause nausea and dizziness.

Licorice Root

Licorice roots are used in aiding digestion, treating upper respiratory problems, and for relieving stress. Licorice works as a muscle relaxant, stimulates mucus production, and exhibits antiviral properties. It may protect LDL from oxidation and may reduce the risk of atherosclerosis. One of the compounds found in licorice, glabridin, is a potent antioxidant.[40] *Warning*: Licorice can raise blood pressure and can cause water retention and loss of potassium.

Fennel and Anise

Both fennel and anise plants have been used to increase milk production, produce menstruation, facilitate birth, alleviate hot flashes, and increase libido. Toxicity problems are rare. In 1970 the Council of Europe proposed no restrictions on fennel oil use; the FDA has approved it for food use.[41, 42]

Nonphytoestrogen Herbs

Red Raspberries

The leaves, bark, and roots of red raspberries are used for PMS and menstrual cramps. The herb helps to decrease menstrual blood flow. *Warning*: Red raspberry leaves may inhibit the absorption of iron.

Goldenseal

The roots and rhizomes of goldenseal are used for just about everything. Goldenseal purportedly boosts the immune system, and it seems there is almost no organ or disease state that is not claimed to benefit from its effects. *Warning*: Do not use for long periods of time. It can cause stomach problems.

Damiana

The leaves of damiana help relieve headaches and increase intestinal contractions. In Mexico the herb is touted as an aphrodesiac. *Warning*: Damiana interferes with iron absorption.

Sarsparilla

The roots are used for regulation of hormones.

Commonly Used Herbs

Ginkgo Biloba

The use of ginkgo biloba is an ancient Chinese therapy. Substantial experimental evidence supports that ginkgo biloba extracts have neuroprotective properties that can help with hypoxia/ischemia, seizure activity, and peripheral nerve damage.[43] One study found that ginseng and ginkgo together had a positive effect on brain circulation. This might be helpful in the geriatric community since brain circulation lessens with age.[44] In another study, 216 patients with Alzheimer's type dementia and multi-infarct dementia were given either a placebo or special extract of ginkgo. The treatment groups showed improvement measured by a number of psychological tests.[45]

St. John's Wort (hypericum perforatum)

St. John's wort has been used for hundreds of years. In Germany it has been licensed for the treatment of relieving anxiety, promoting sleep, and elevating spirits. Out of three million patients taking St. John's wort in Germany, few side effects were reported. The known side effects are gastrointestinal symptoms, allergic reactions, and fatigue.[46] The herb has been effective for positively treating depression when compared with a placebo. It has effects similar to standard antidepressants.[47]

31

Menopause

Natural menopause has technically arrived when menstruation has ceased for one year. Surgical menopause occurs abruptly at the time of surgery, when ovaries are removed. The climacteric is that period of years during which the body uses the last of its eggs and hormonal changes begin to occur. As the number of eggs decrease, the levels of estrogen and progesterone produced by the ovaries begin to fluctuate. The pituitary no longer perceives the higher, premenopausal levels of hormones and works harder to promote them. It raises the follicle stimulating hormone (FSH) as much as 13 times and raises the luteinizing hormone (LH) levels 3 times in its attempt to stimulate the ovaries to release eggs. Eventually, without ovulation, estrogen levels drop, progesterone production ceases, the uterine lining does not thicken, and menstruation stops. After menopause has occurred, estrogen is made from androstenedione, a weak male hormone produced in the ovaries and adrenal glands, and converted into estrogen by fat, liver, and kidney tissues.[1,2]

Menstruation may end gradually, abruptly, or erratically. In the United States, 10 percent of women go through menopause by age 38, 30 percent by age 44, 50 percent by age 49, 90 percent by age 54, and 100 percent by age 58. Women who are thin, smoke cigarettes, have had twins, have had less education, and have lower incomes tend to experience menopause earlier than other women.[3]

With menopause, many women experience hot flashes, headaches, sleeplessness, mood swings, vertigo, heart palpitations, shortness of breath, asthma, fatigue, libido changes, and digestive problems. Internally the vagina can change from being moist and reddish in color to dry and pale. The cervix changes from being soft to firm. The breasts may change: Smaller breasts tend to become smaller and flatter. Larger breasts tend to elongate and droop. The nipples become smaller and may lose their ability to become erect.[4] The bladder and urethra lose muscle tone and decrease their production of fluids that help to ward off infection.[5] (See Chapter 33.) Unfelt initially but eventually more important are losses in bone mass, which may lead to osteoporosis.

The good news is that birth control problems are solved, and women who suffered with PMS find that problem alleviated. Women who stop menstruating abruptly either naturally or surgically tend to have more problems than women who go through the hormonal changes more gradually. Also, thin women tend to have more acute problems than heavier women. A sudden drop in the estrogen level or low estrogen reserves accompanying low body fat appears to amplify the discomforts.

Every woman experiences the "change of life" differently. Up to 10 to 15 percent of women slide through these years not noticing any difficulties, and 10 to 15 percent are severely debilitated.[6] However, the majority of women have at least a few bothersome problems.

Hot flashes occur in up to 85 percent of women and are very troublesome for 10 to 20 percent. They can disrupt sleep night after night, leaving a woman exhausted and worn down. When a hot flash occurs, the skin temperature rises 4 to 8 degrees Fahrenheit, due to capillary dilatation, and the body temperature drops.[7] Hot flashes generally occur for about two years; and in a small number of cases, they can persist up to ten years or more.

When the levels of estrogen drop, the mucous membranes, skin, and urogenital tissues are affected. The skin loses its moisture, and the vaginal mucosa can become thin and dry, resulting in painful intercourse. There also can be a thinning and drying of the urethral (urine canal) tissues, causing painful urination, problems with incontinence, and an increase in urinary tract infections.

Some women find that they have an increased libido (sexual desire), some notice it decreased, and some notice no change at all. Androgens are major contributors that can affect sexual interest and desire. During the climacteric and postmenopausally, there is a drop in estrogen levels but a plateau in testosterone levels. Some researchers have attributed elevated libido to higher testosterone levels. Decreased libido can occur in women who have had oophorectomies, or removal of the ovaries, since the ovaries produce androgen as well as estrogen. However, we are not totally ruled by our hormones. A woman's feelings about sex, herself, her partner, and the world around her strongly influence her interest and desire for sex.[8, 9]

With the thinning, shrinking, and drying of the vagina, sexual activity may be less comfortable. It may take longer to produce enough fluids for penetration. Lubricants may be necessary. There also may be a less pronounced sexual sensation due to decreased blood flow to the vaginal area.

Mood swings may also be produced by the drops and fluctuations of estrogen and progesterone levels. Lowered estrogen levels also are known to cause sleep disturbances.

The following are different treatments that have been used for menopausal problems:

- Hormone replacement therapy (HRT—for women with a uterus) and estrogen therapy (ERT—for women without a uterus) relieve many of the problems associated with midlife and menopausal complaints. ERT and HRT have been shown to reduce or completely stop hot flashes, reduce bone loss, and possibly reduce the risk of heart disease. However, these therapies have side effects. They are not for everybody.
- Estrogen cream may also be helpful in relieving vaginal dryness.
- Testosterone creams have been said to increase a woman's libido. However, these may have masculinizing effects. (See also Chapter 25.)
- Progesterone cream, along with a good diet and exercise, relieves most menopausal complaints for many women. Menopausal women not using an estrogen supplement would apply the progesterone cream for 14 to 21 days per month. Women supplementing with estrogen would use the progesterone cream for 21 to 25 days each month.

Alternatives to ERT and HRT[10, 11]

Women for whom ERT or HRT is contraindicated have a few alternatives available to them. However, there is no clear treatment consensus. Each woman needs to be assessed regarding her own medical status and current medications. In a 1996 study, postmenopausal women who did not take estrogen replacement had an increased natural killer cell activity. This natural killer cell activity is decreased during estrogen substitution. Natural killer cells play an important role in the nonadaptive immune system, defend against viral infections, and are involved in tumor surveillance. The natural killer cell activity is inversely related to the development of neoplasms, viral infections, and the spread of metastatic disease.[12]

Stop smoking! Smoking makes hot flashes more severe,[13] increases your risk of heart disease, cancer, osteoporosis, and lung disease; and shortens your life span.

Vitamin E has been used for relieving hot flashes. Some people have suggested taking 1,000 IU per day of vitamin E either with or without 500 mg of vitamin C, and 25 mcg of selenium. Check with a physician if you have high blood pressure or are taking digitalis. (See Chapter 7.)

Vitamin A supplementation has been used for vaginal dryness.

Do not let your body fat drop below 15 percent. This reduces the amount of estrogen in your body. A little fat is in.

Take care of your heart. Eat more vegetables and fruits high in beta-carotene, polyunsaturated fats, fish, soybeans, whole grains, and less meat. Postmenopausally reduce iron intake and eliminate it from supplementation. Check with your physician. (See Chapter 29.)

Megestrol acetate or medroxyprogesterone acetate may provide significant relief from menopausal discomforts.

Clonidine (a blood pressure medication) and medroxyprogesterone may be an alternative if the side effects can be tolerated.[14]

Selective estrogen receptor modulators (SERMS) work by mimicking certain effects of estrogen. Yet they have the ability to send or not send signals to different organs in the body. For example, tamoxifen, sometimes used for breast cancer, binds to breast estrogen receptors and blocks estrogen. The different SERMS have different jobs. SERMS can produce either estrogen agonist or estrogen antagonist effects.

Raloxifene (Evista[15]), which appears to have an improved safety profile, is an alternative to ERT or HRT in postmenopausal women for the prevention and treatment of osteoporosis and cardiovascular disease without many of the side effects of ERT/HRT.[16] Pending further studies, raloxifene may also prove to be useful in preventing breast cancer. The role of SERMs looks bright for the future.

Women with low risk of osteoporosis or heart disease can take nutritional and biological phytoestrogens with oral or topical micronized progesterone to reduce menopausal complaints. Women in the high-risk group can take plant-derived conventional oral, transdermal, or natural estrogens along with micronized progesterone.

Estriol has been touted as the estrogen choice by many. It is the predominant estrogen produced by the placenta. It has been suggested that estriol protects against breast and endometrial cancers. It has a very low biological activity and binds to estrogen receptors with one-third to one-half of estradiol. Studies have shown that women who have children early produce more estriol than women who have never had children. Also, Asian women have higher levels of estriol than American women.

Ginseng, licorice, fenugreek, sarsaparilla, gota kola, wild Mexican yam, and dong quai are reputed as having estrogenic activity. (See Chapter 30.)

Wild yam contains a small amount of DHEA and produces sterols, called saponins, which are similar to progesterone. (See Chapter 30.) Wild yam promotes the production of progesterone, reduces menopausal symptoms and improves libido, and may increase bone density. It has been suggested that progesterone cream applied directly to tender or lumpy breasts may reduce the conditions.

Dehydroepiandrosterone (DHEA) is a steroid-hormone that has been said to improve the immune system, slow aging, increase energy, improve lipids, improve mood and libido, and may have a protective effect against cancer.[17] DHEA is converted into androgens, including testosterone, androstenedione, and dihydrotestosterone. DHEA is quite low until puberty, increases and peaks at age 25, and declines until approximately age 70.[18] DHEA has been shown to increase natural killer cells, increase androgen levels, and increases muscle strength.[19, 20]

DHEA has been used frequently in the past few years. Side effects that may be associated with high doses and long-term use are still unknown. Side effects include hirsutism, voice deepening, and decreased HDL cholesterol. Nausea, vomiting, seborrheic dermatitis, and jaundice are seen with low-dose chronic use.[21]

Approximately 2 ounces of tofu daily has been shown to effectively reduce hot flashes, decrease natural dryness, and assist in maintaining bone density. Phytoestrogen-rich diets, 45 mg per day, affect the hormonal status and exert a significant physiological effect on the regulation of the menstrual cycle. Japanese subjects consume on average 50 to 100 mg of isoflavones per day from soy products. The average plasma estradiol values of postmenopausal women in Western societies are in the range of 15 to 30 picogram (pg) per ml. Thus the phytoestrogen levels may exceed those of endogenous estradiol by a thousandfold.[22] (See Chapter 30.)

Start exercising or continue to exercise. Exercise may help to lessen severity of hot flashes. Exercise also reduces the risk of heart disease and osteoporosis and reduces stress that may be associated with hormonal changes. (See Chapter 26.)

Vaginal lubricants such as K-Y Jelly, vegetable oil, saliva, and massage oils can be helpful for vaginal dryness.

Feed your bones. It has been recommended by many physicians and researchers to supplement your diet with 1,000 mg of calcium premenopausally and 1,500 mg postmenopausally. Include in your supplement vitamin K, magnesium, manganese, boron, phosphorus, and zinc.

32

Premenstrual Syndrome (PMS)

PREMENSTRUAL SYNDROME (PMS) has a wide range of symptoms that recur monthly. Seventy-five percent of menstruating women have some physical, emotional, or behavioral symptoms premenstrually. Only 3 to 8 percent of menstruating women have extremely severe symptoms. This severe form of premenstrual syndrome is called premenstrual dysphoria disorder (PMDD). Premenstrual magnification (PMM) occurs when premenstrual symptoms are concurrent with psychiatric disorders. Each of these forms of premenstrual disorder has its own strict criteria that do not overlap.

The syndromes have been attributed to normal ovarian function, triggering cyclical biochemical changes in the brain, rather than a hormonal imbalance as once believed. However, the exact cause of the syndromes are unknown, as are the remedies. Although no cure exists for PMS, PMM, and PMDD, some recommendations to reduce many of the symptoms are available. General remedies include limiting certain foods and eating others, vitamin and mineral supplementation, exercise, and reduction of stress. Some medical treatments include hormonal and psychoactive agents.

Ruling out other medical disorders such as hypoglycemia (low blood sugar), thyroid problems, and manic depression is important. Each of these disorders presents many of the same symptoms as PMS.

In the case of hypoglycemia, it is important to have the blood sugar levels drawn during the premenstruum.[1]

Foods that should be avoided are sugar, processed foods, refined carbohydrates, caffeine, alcohol, and salt. Foods that may help include complex carbohydrates, fruits, and vegetables. It is also advisable to eat many small meals per day rather than a few larger ones and drink plenty of water. However, be sure to maintain the total caloric intake. Exercise is essential to alleviate stress and enhance general health.

Although supplementation of B_6 (pyridoxine) has been used as a treatment for PMS, its value has been disputed. In one study on premenstrual anxiety, irritability, and nervous tension, the symptoms of PMS were reduced when the women were given 200 to 800 mg per day of B_6. It was noted that the women in this study had high levels of estrogen and low levels of progesterone; 200 to 800 mg of B_6 reduced the estrogen levels and increased the progesterone levels. It was also reported that B_6 reduced water retention problems by lowering aldosterone (a kidney-regulating hormone) levels.[2] In another double-blind, placebo study, similar results were found. Twenty-one of twenty-five women with PMS receiving 500 mg of B_6 per day for a three-month period experienced fewer symptoms of PMS.[3] However, chronic vitamin B_6 supplementation has been shown to be toxic at low doses. In one study, more than 100 women taking an average of 117 mg of B_6 per day for six months to five years reported neurological symptoms. When the supplementation of B_6 was stopped, the women completely recovered from their symptoms within six months.[4]

Lethargy and muscle weakness occurring throughout the cycle may be attributed to a depletion of potassium, especially if diuretics have been used. During the premenstrual period, sodium and water are retained in the body and potassium is reduced through urination. Potassium supplementation or extra servings of fruits and vegetables, but not juices, may be helpful to relieve these symptoms.[5,6] (See Chapter 20.)

According to reports, many of the most common complaints of PMS may be attributed to magnesium deficiency. Magnesium deficiency causes a drop in brain dopamine levels without a commensurate drop in norepinephrine or serotonin, causing anxiety and depressive symptoms.[7] (Dopamine, norepinephrine, and serotonin are all nerve messenger chemicals in the brain.) Also, chocolate cravings may be an indication of a magnesium deficiency.[8] A magnesium to calcium ratio of 2 to 1 may relieve many of the symptoms of PMS.[9] It is generally accepted that the magnesium to calcium ratio is approximately 1 to almost 3. The magnesium/calcium balance is a critical factor in preserving bone density. (See Chapters 11 and 23.)

One treatment of PMS is natural progesterone. It is important to note that natural progesterone and synthetic progestogens are not equivalent agents. Synthetic progestogens do not have exactly the same effects on the body as natural progesterone does and generally result in more side effects.[10,11] Natural progesterone treatments may be administered by injection, pill, suppository, or cream. Natural progesterone cream containing approximately 480 mg per ounce has been shown to beneficially affect most PMS symptoms when applied as directed. At this level there are no known side effects. The use of natural progesterone therapy has been an accepted treatment for PMS in Britain for many years. No major side effects were reported over a 30-year period with the use of the therapy.[12]

Another common treatment for PMS is estradiol. Both estradiol implants and transdermal estradiol suppress ovulation. It is not known if the reduction of symptoms of PMS is due to the disruption of the menstrual cycle or due to suppression of ovulation. However, as opposed to naturally occurring estradiol, *conjugated estrogens* have been shown to exacerbate the symptoms.[13]

Other hormonal treatments include danazol, leuprolide, and oral contraceptives. Although these are purported to relieve the symptoms of PMS, they are not free of side effects.[14] Another often prescribed treatment, tranquilizers, can be effective, but may lead to abuse.

Researchers found that the following therapy can help relieve PMS:

B6—100 mg daily
Calcium—1,000 mg daily
Magnesium—360 mg daily (luteal phase only)
Vitamin E—400 IU daily
Tryptophan—6 g daily (luteal phase only)
Vitamin supplementation
Bright artificial lights—one-half to one hour treatment at 10,000 lux at 7 P.M. daily (luteal week)

Positive thinking[15]
Natural progesterone cream—20–30 mg per day (luteal phase only, days 12–26 of menstrual cycle)

Women who meet the criteria for PMDD can be treated successfully with selective serotonin reuptake inhibitors (SSRIs) such as Prozac, Zoloft, and gonadotropin-releasing hormone agonists (GnRH-a) drugs. The SSRIs are antidepressants and GnRH-as suppress ovarian function.[16,17] SSRI's side effects are reduced libido, inability to have an orgasm, sweating, and vertigo.[18] They also have a tendency to lose their effectiveness in a relatively short amount of time.[19] Fluoxetine has been an effective treatment of PMDD.[20] GnRH-a side effects are menopausal-like, including night sweats and hot flashes. Although both of these treatments have been found effective, they do not work on all women.

Women who meet the criteria for PMM need to be treated by a physician that specializes in both PMS and psychiatric disorders.

In all three cases—PMS, PMM, and PMDD, check with your physician. New medications become available all the time.

We recommend reading *What Your Doctor May Not Tell You About Menopause* by Dr. John R. Lee and Virginia Hopkins.

33

Skin and Aging

THE SKIN PERFORMS a number of functions critical to health and well-being. The *epidermis* (the outside layer of the skin) prevents fluid loss and protects the lower levels of skin from physical insults of the outside world as well as from microorganisms. With the help of melanin (skin pigment), the epidermis protects us against the carcinogenic effects of ultraviolet radiation. The *dermis* (the inner layer of the skin) controls body temperature by increasing or decreasing the blood flow through the skin's circulatory system and by regulating the activity of the sweat glands. The *subcutis* (subcutaneous fat, the bottom layer of the skin) serves as padding to protect the organs beneath, as well as providing insulation and energy storage. The total weight of all bodily skin on an adult is estimated at 7 to 9 pounds with an area of 20 square feet. The skin is the largest organ of the body.[1]

Epidermis

The epidermis, or outer layer of skin, contains several layers of cells: the stratum corneum—a dead, horny, surface layer made up largely of the protein keratin—and the deeper layers of live cells. These are the granular, spinous, and basal cell layers. The layers of skin vary in thickness depending on location. For example, the epidermis is very thick on the palms and soles, but is very thin in the vagina and on the eyelids. The epidermis develops from the basal cells on its deep aspect. The basal cell layer, by cell division, produces a constant supply of new skin cells, which mature into flat, tough, keratin-filled, platelike cells that form the horny, dry skin surface. This outer layer is continuously sloughed off, leaving newer skin cells showing. The entire growth of the skin from the basal layer to the epidermal surface takes approximately one month. If this process is not interrupted by any extraneous influences, it will produce smooth and pliable skin.

Two functional rather than structural cell types are found in the epidermis: the melanocyte and the Langerhan's cell. *Melanocytes* derive from the same embryonic tissue that gives rise to brain and nerves. However, these specialized cells produce a pigment called melanin, which gives us our distinct skin and hair colors. These are variations of yellow, brown, and red. Our own genetic makeup determines what our skin and hair colors will be. Melanin is an excellent absorber of ultraviolet light. The denser the melanin, the darker the skin color and the more built-in protection from the sun.

The *Langerhan's cells* are derived from the bone marrow and play a role in the skin's immunology. These cells can capture and process antigenic materials that come in contact with the skin and eliminate them through the lymphatic system. They are decisive in determining immunity, tolerance, or allergy to various substances.

Dermis

The dermis, or lower skin, is also thick or thin depending on the specific region of the body. For example, the dermis is very thick on the back but very thin on the palms. This lower skin layer is made up of collagen and elastin set in a web of jellylike matrix (glycosaminoglycans). The elastin fibers are intertwined with the collagen and are the main reason why skin is elastic. The glycosaminoglycans act like a sponge holding water. This material controls how much moisture our skin contains. Within the collagen-elastin network is a maze of blood vessels, nerves, sweat glands, ducts, and lymphatics. The nerve sensors enable us to feel touch, pressure, temperature, and pain. Oil glands, or sebaceous glands, which are largest and most numerous on the face, chest, scalp, and back, produce many different fats and waxes. This mixture of fats and waxes, called *sebum*, is secreted from the oil gland into a duct or hair follicle and moves from there to the skin surface. Sebum lubricates the skin and protects it from drying out.

Pores are the openings to sweat and oil glands located in lower skin layers. The size of the pores is mostly determined by heredity and age.

Subcutis

The subcutis, a subcutaneous fat layer, protects the organs beneath and is a storage area for energy and nutrients. It is thought that the quantity of fat cells is largely determined by heredity. This layer houses the apocrine glands and the eccrine glands. *Apocrine glands* are usually found in the armpits, areolae (skin around nipple), around the belly button, and in the genital and anal regions. They produce milky sweat that is secreted into the upper section of the hair follicle and is eliminated to the skin surface. This secretion is attacked by bacteria and causes body odor. The *eccrine glands* are common sweat glands. They have ducts to transport sweat directly to the surface. Sweat consists of water and a few salts, is odorless, and is produced in response to exercise, heat, stress, and fevers. It cools the body by evaporation.

Aging Skin

Many of the skin changes that happen in our 30s, 40s and 50s are wrongly blamed on menopause. Most of these changes, the wrinkles (our character lines) and spots, are due to aging, heredity, cigarette smoking, sun damage, and other environmental factors. When we are young, the skin growth cycle may take as little time as two weeks. However, between the third and seventh decade, 50 percent decrease in the cell turnover rate occurs.[2]

In young children, prior to significant sun exposure, the skin has an orderly geometric pattern. The epidermis has a network of infolding ridges that reach down into the dermis. These form a geography of plateaus and crisscrossing valleys at the interface between the dermis and epidermis, resulting in an increase in surface area at that interface. In aged skin, the overall geometry remains the same, but the entire epidermis is thinner, decreasing approximately 20 percent in thickness over one's lifetime.[3] The rete ridges disappear and diminish the area of contact between the dermis and the epidermis. The valleys are shallower and the plateaus are larger. The epidermal turnover rate is decreased by 30 to 50 percent. This results in slower skin growth and is a possible reason why older folks don't heal as well as younger ones. Both the melanocytes and the Langerhan's cells appear decreased in number as we age, and the pores tend to become larger. Presently, no products are on the market that really will shrink the pores for more than a few hours.[4]

In the skin of a small child, the fine collagen bundles are in a simple pattern parallel to the skin's surface. In older skin, the collagen bundles are tightly packed and are randomly oriented. Collagen is thought to decrease up to 1 percent a year during adult life.[5] Whether there is a gradual or rapid loss of glycosaminoglycans is in dispute. One theory suggests a loss of glycosaminoglycans and a flattening of collagen occurs, resulting in the filling of empty spaces and crowding of elastin fibers.[6] Consequently, there is thinning of the dermal layer and a loss of resiliency of the skin and its ability to retain water. Elastin fibers decrease in numbers, unravel, fragment, and straighten, which results in a loss of elasticity.[7] A decrease in circulation and in the function of the sweat glands also occurs. Women have an estimated 32 percent reduction per decade in the sebum (oil) production after the age of 20.[8] As a result, our skin becomes drier as we age.

Premature Aging

Sun Damage

Skin that has been exposed to the sun one too many times has distinctly different physical characteristics than nonexposed skin. Women who have had a life of sun exposure look older than women who have had little sun exposure.[9] The most obvious effects are increased wrinkling, uneven pigmentation, and increased risk of cancer.

The skin first loses its geometric pattern, which may result in cracking and fissuring.[10] The melanin in our skin acts as a sunscreen, but through years of exposure to the sun, the pigment cells become damaged and lose their protective ability. Melanocytes are two to three times as numerous in exposed skin as in nonexposed skin.[11] The increase in the number and density of the groupings of the melanocytes alternating with areas of loss creates age spots and uneven tanning. A loss of pigment cells through the natural aging process only compounds the problem for future sun exposure. This melanocyte loss and damage leaves us less protected, adding to the direct assault of the ultraviolet rays on our skin. In the dermal layer, the collagen fibers have a decreased resiliency and the elastin fibers turn into shapeless, fuzzy clumps.[12] These changes leave a blotchy, cancer-prone skin with a leathery, nonelastic texture.

Skin Cancer

In the United States, more than 600,000 cases of basal cell and squamous cell skin cancers are diagnosed yearly. Most of these cases are thought to be related to sun exposure. Fortunately both cancers have a high cure rate.

It is also strongly suspected that melanomas are related to solar radiation.[13] There were 15,000 cases reported in women in 1992; an estimated 2,600 women in the United States will die this year from melanomas. More cases are reported near the equator, and people with lighter skin color are more susceptible.[14]

Smoking

Tobacco smoking damages collagen and impairs the blood circulation to the skin. Constriction of blood vessels results in a decrease in nutrients and oxygen delivered to the various layers of skin. The result is yellowish skin color, cross-hatched wrinkles on the face, a lot of tiny and not so tiny lines all around the mouth, and crow's feet by the eyes. Cigarette smoking is also estimated to be responsible for 79 percent of lung cancer in women and for 30 percent of all cancer deaths.[15] Remember, smoking is *the* leading cause of cancer deaths in women.

Heat, Cold, and Weight Loss

People exposed to extreme temperatures in their environment or in the sauna are more likely to wrinkle. The temperature extremes put extra stress on the skin. People who lose weight may have a problem with cutaneous elasticity, causing extra wrinkles and skin that tends to sag. Sometimes skin is not resilient enough to follow the new shape of the body.[16]

"Spots and Things"—(and what to do about them)

Seborrheic Keratoses

Seborrheic keratoses are harmless, hard or scaley, black, brown, or gray spots on the skin. They are often velvety, rough, or warty. They may be removed by liquid nitrogen, electrodesiccation, or surgery. One must remember that, depending on the site, size, and removal technique, the treatment may leave a scar that is more noticeable than the spot.

Actinic Keratoses

Actinic keratosis, are caused by chronic sun exposure, are rough, scaly, and usually pinkish or reddish-brown. They are precancerous and should be treated. Depending on the location, size, and thickness, treatment may involve liquid nitrogen, electrodesiccation, acid application, dermabrasion, curettage, or treatment with a chemotherapy cream.

Basal Cell Carcinomas

Basal cell carcinomas are common, raised, bumpy, or flat spots that may bleed, scale, and sometimes be confused with pimples. Basal cell skin cancers need to be treated. Although they can cause extensive local destruction if not treated when small, they have no significant tendency to metastasize, or spread.

Squamous Cell Carcinomas

Another common form of skin cancer, squamous cell carcinomas are bumpy, scaly, crusted, or warty pinkish growths that tend to bleed and become inflamed. These may metastasize throughout the body, although it is uncommon.

Malignant Melanomas

The most serious and least common of the major skin cancers, malignant melanomas may resemble moles, be flat or raised, but usually have irregular or indistinct borders. As they develop, their color may change to include blue, black, red, tan, white, and brown. Any new or recently changed mole or pigmented spot is suspect. Any spot with multiple colors or irregular color distribution is suspect. Any spot or mole with irregular borders is suspect. Treatment is simple and curative if the cancer is diagnosed early, but the cancer is often fatal if detected late.

Spider Veins (Telangiectases)

The tiny veins that mostly appear on the legs or cheeks are nothing more than prominent superficial capillaries. These veins are near the surface of the skin, supplying neither nutrition nor oxygen to the areas. Spider veins may be removed for cosmetic reasons by electrodesiccation, sclerotherapy, or laser treatments.

Cherry Spots (Cherry Angiomas, Senile Angiomas)

Cherry spots are usually small, raised, red spots that appear on the skin more and more frequently with age. They are harmless but may be bothersome cosmetically or physically, depending on location. They are quite easy to remove with liquid nitrogen or electrodesiccation.

Skin Tags

Skin tags are small, harmless extra flaps of skin that may be annoying. Women over age 40 and postmenopausal women are prone to grow them. There is also a familial predisposition. They usually appear around the neck, eyelids, groins, armpits, and shoulders. These can be removed by electrosurgery or liquid nitrogen.

Moles (Nevi)

Generally, moles are harmless. They can be flat or raised and are usually brown, tan, or pink. However, they should be watched carefully for any irregularity or changes in size, color, texture, or border shape, as well as any tendency to bleeding or inflammation. These changes may herald a change into a melanoma (cancer) and need to be checked by a dermatologist.

Cysts

Sebaceous glands in the dermis and subcutaneous fat sometimes form a sac filled with a harmless cheese-like substance. Usually, a large pore leads to the skin surface. So-called sebaceous cysts are frequently found on the back, scalp, or face and range in size from a small bean to a Ping-Pong ball. On the head they are commonly called wens and often cause bald spots on the overlying scalp due to chronic pressure impeding blood flow to the hair follicles. Occasionally cysts become inflamed and swell up like boils. Cysts can be removed surgically if inflamed or uncomfortable or for cosmetic reasons.

Age Spots or Liver Spots (Senile Lentigines)

It might be preferable to call age spots by their literal translation, "freckles of old age." Changes in pigmentation due to clustering of melanocytes, they are large dark spots and are harmless. Bleaching creams will reduce the color over a few months, but the spots will return if the area is exposed to the sun. Liquid nitrogen, chemical formulas, cryotherapy, and electrosurgery are used to remove the spots. Once again, scarring or white spots may be more noticeable than the initial lesion.

Sun Damage Prevention, Treatments, and Procedures

Treatments and skin care products are available that will rejuvenate some of the damaged skin, but the best answer is to avoid sun damage to begin with. All of us will have some wrinkles eventually, but healthy and attractive skin is possible despite them.

Use a good sunscreen with a sun protection factor (SPF) of 15. Sunscreens with SPFs of 30 or above may actually cause dryness problems due to the higher concentrations of the chemicals in the sunscreen. Presently many good sunscreens are available. There are gels and creams for the sports-minded or those who perspire heavily; these agents will persist for hours unless you use soap. There are sunscreens for use under your makeup, in your makeup, and as moisturizers. There are sunscreens with para-aminobenzoic acid (PABA) and without. (As many as 5 percent of people get allergies to PABA.) Whether or not you use makeup, it is a good idea to get in the habit of applying some form of a sunscreen in the morning as a protective shield. Just protecting your skin from the sun will allow your skin to heal itself to some degree and will also deter further damage. If you really want a tan, try some of the new skin-staining products. Chemically based rather than radiation based, they will give your skin a darker color.

There is an ongoing controversy concerning the possibility that sunscreens are worthless or actually harmful when it comes to preventing skin cancers. The gist of the argument is that most sunscreens efficiently screen out short-range ultraviolet (UVB) light but do a lousy job of screening long-range ultraviolet (UVA) light. This does prevent acute sunburns, but it allows a person who would normally stay out in the sun 20 minutes (and accumulate 20 minutes worth of UVA damage) to stay out 5 hours (and accumulate 5 hours of UVA damage). So the worry is that sunscreens enable a lot of people to suffer a lot more UVA injury than they could without sunscreens. This is not good since UVA is suspected to cause both aging changes and skin cancers. However, some of the newer sunscreens efficiently filter both UVA and UVB. One type contains microscopically powdered titanium dioxide, which acts as a physical barrier to all wavelengths. The other contains newer chemical sunscreens active in the UVA range. In light of current evidence, the best recommdations are to use a full-spectrum UVA/UVB sunscreen and to use it as a protection, not an excuse to abuse your skin with ever longer hours in the sun.

It has been suggested that sun damage may be mitigated by supplementing the diet with 400 IU of vitamin E as d-alpha tocopherol acetate and 100 mcg of selenium. For immediate relief, taking approximately 2,000 IU of vitamin E along with one or two aspirins will help alleviate a sunburn and its inflammation. The vitamin E must be taken soon after the sun exposure.[17] But in light of other reports that the damage done by radiation may depend on the total antioxidant pool in the body, it is probably prudent to balance all the antioxidant vitamins.

Whether or not you use sunscreens or take antioxidants, wear clothes that will protect you from the sun, including dark polarized sunglasses, a wide brimmed hat, and long sleeves.

Tretinoin, known as Retin-A,[18] is a vitamin A derivative. This drug has received a tremendous amount of attention since 1988. It was almost exclusively used to treat acne before it was reported to rejuvenate sun-damaged skin. It makes the skin more youthful-looking by removing the top layers of dead skin scales, plumping out fine wrinkles, and fading much of the blotchy, brown pigmentation that accompanies photoaging. In addition, Retin-A appears to repair some of the damage done to the skin's blood vessels and to incite production of new, healthy collagen over old, sun-damaged collagen. Side affects may include skin irritation and an increased susceptibility to sunburn, windburn, and winter chapping. The FDA has not approved the use of Retin-A for wrinkles. It has, however, approved Renova[19] for the treatment of wrinkles. Renova is really tretinoin reformulated in a new base that is friendlier to dry, sun-damaged, older skin.

Two new drugs, Vivida[20] and Imedeen,[21] are both treatments for sun-damaged skin that are derived from cartilage of marine fish. European studies have purported to show that treated skin is thicker, has a smoother appearance, and appears to have greater elasticity. The only side effects reported were pimples in the first few weeks of use. Brittleness of both the hair and nails were also reported to improve with treatment.[22]

Acid peels are commonly employed procedures for rejuvenating facial skin. They can generally be divided into three classes: light, medium, and deep. As with most things, you get what you pay for. In the case of acid peels, the payment is an increase in risk and pain for deeper peels in return for the promise of more dramatic rejuvenating changes.

Light peels affect only the epidermis. The dermis remains unscathed. This means that only superficial blemishes confined to the epidermis can be treated, including keratoses, many pigmentation problems, and dull, dry skin texture. Wrinkles and scars are not affected by light peels. The advantage is that they are safe since the dermis is not injured. A variety of agents including Retin-A, trichloroacetic acid, and the alpha-hydroxy acids such as glycolic acid are used. Light peels may or may not result in redness and peeling, depending on the agent used. Recovery, however, is quick, at most only a few days. And in general, no time need be lost from your general routine. These peels give an immediate improvement in appearance and texture, but some experienced clinicians feel that, at the end of a year's time, there is not much difference to be seen between faces treated with in-office glycolic acid peels and faces treated daily at home with a good glycolic acid moisturizer.

Medium-depth peels wound the epidermis and the uppermost dermis. This means that some minor wrinkles can be eradicated, in addition to resurfacing the epidermis. In general, the same agents are used as in light peels, but at greater concentrations or for longer exposure times. The recovery times are also consequently longer, and rawness or sheetlike shedding of the facial skin is the rule.

Deep peels wound the dermis relatively deeply. The epidermis is obliterated. Controlled healing results in reorganization of the skin collagen similar to remolding plastic after melting it. Numerous agents are used, but the gold standard of deep peels is the phenol peel. Expertly used, the deep peel is capable of effacing even moderately deep lines and wrinkles and is often used to get rid of the radiating furrows that develop around the mouth. Scarring is a hazard, as is the loss of natural skin pigment in the treated areas, sometimes leaving the patient with a ghostly appearance unless makeup is worn. Cardiac monitoring is routinely done with phenol peels because of the reported heart toxicity of phenol. Recovery is prolonged, and sun avoidance for 6 to 12 months is often required to prevent pigment blotching.

Dermabrasion is a technique that uses high-speed rotating wire brushes or diamond fraises to literally sand away your wrinkles. This procedure may produce scarring, mottled pigmentation, and uneven healing of the skin just as deep peels do. This also must be performed by a physician.

Collagen injections are used to fill in wrinkles and scars by injecting a creamy preparation of purified cow collagen into the dermis. This is a temporary treatment since the bovine collagen is gradually metabolized by the body. Touch-up injections must be done every few months to maintain any cosmetic improvement. Allergies to the injected materials may result.

Liposuction is the process of removing fat from subcutaneous areas to change a specific contour of the body.

Microlipoinjection (fat transplantation) is the technique of removing fat, usually from the abdomen, thighs, or buttocks, and using it to fill in scars or wrinkles. The fat is extracted with a large bore needle, rinsed of blood, and reinjected into the target site. It is a temporary treatment that has the best success if used in places where there is little skin movement.[23]

Blepharoplasties (eyelid tucks) and facial rhytidectomies (face-lifts) are techniques used to surgically remove sagging and wrinkles.

Among the most promising new cosmetic procedures is laser resurfacing. Diffusing the beam of a laser changes it from a tool that cuts and punches holes to an instrument that can peel very thin layers off the skin surface. Resurfacing the skin with a laser does much the same thing as an acid peel or dermabrasion. Depending on the type of laser and the technique, the peel can vary from extremely superficial to moderately deep, with the consequent range of healing times, risk, and cosmetic improvement. A distinct advantage of resurfacing with certain types of lasers is that the skin collagen shortens considerably—about 30 percent—due to the heat produced in the skin. This results in a substantial tightening of loose, sagging skin in addition to the cosmetic improvement of renewing the skin surface, eliminating lines, wrinkles, and pigment irregularities. (See Susan Roper's article at the end of this chapter.)

New moisturizer formulations have been big news for the past few years, and with good reason: The alpha-hydroxy acid moisturizers available now are the only truly new technology in moisturizers for the past century. (Glycolic acid is undoubtably the most flexible and effective of the choices, but several others are used for their particular characteristics.) Traditional moisturizers are almost all emulsions of oil and water in different ratios with a variety of modifying agents. But they all do the same thing. They put a little water into the skin and cover it with oil to retard evaporation. After a few hours, the oil wears off or evaporates, then the water evaporates, too, leaving the skin in about the same state it was before. On the other hand, alpha-hydroxy acid moisturizers peel away dry scale on the surface. The remaining scale is transformed into a compact rather than open-weave pattern, which is efficient at retaining the skin's own moisture. Long-term use also appears to result in the development of new, healthy collagen fibers in the upper dermis. Overall, the effect is really a mild rejuvenation, which has led to a paradox for cosmetic companies. For years, they advertised oil and water moisturizers with false claims of rejuvenating powers. Now the industry finally has something that actually delivers on the promise, but it can't directly say so in its advertising. If companies claim that their products truly rejuvenate the skin, then the FDA can declare them drugs and regulate them as such, moving them away from the cosmetic industry. So now the advertising has to tiptoe around the truth instead of inching up to a lie.

Nails

The nail consists of dead, cornified cells that are produced by the nail matrix. The matrix, or nail bud, is located under the cuticle and extends a short distance out under the nail. The only visible area of the matrix is the lunula, or whitish moon that can be seen in your nail. The nail itself, properly called the nail plate, is made of many layers of tightly bonded platelets of nonliving substance produced by the matrix. Most of the substance in the nail is keratin, which is the same protein that makes up the skin surface and hair. Much of the flexibility of the nails is dependent upon the water content of the nail. This hydration is in turn dependent on the relative humidity.

The growth of our nails increases in our 20s and 30s and appears to decrease after that as people age. Fingernails grow about 0.1 to 0.25 inch a month, and toenails grow about half as fast. The nails grow faster in the summer months than they do in the winter or in colder climates. With age may come irregularity of nail growth.[24,25] Ridges and uneven growth patterns occur. However, most complaints that are heard from 40- to 60-year-old women are of brittle nails. This change may occur suddenly around or sometime after menopause. When this happens, the nails remain brittle for about four years and then improve. There does not seem to be any treatment that helps to relieve this problem but time.[26]

Another nail problem that occurs more frequently with age is fungal infection of the toenails, especially on the large toes. This results in thick, dull, discolored, and often deformed and uncomfortable nails. Unfortunately, no topical agents reliably treat this problem. Several new and effective oral medications have been advertised heavily in the media. These drugs do work well and treatment usually will result in normal nails. However, the drugs must be taken over a period of months, are expensive, have interactions with numerous other common medications, and do not prevent later reinfection. This last item is a real problem if you have toenail fungus or athlete's foot, since every one of your shoes is impregnated with fungal spores that pose a reinfection risk. The expense of replacing your entire shoe wardrobe varies from considerable to staggering.

The majority of cases of toenail fungus can probably be avoided in the first place by wearing shoes that fit properly. The hypothesis has been convincingly advanced that fungus infections occur almost exclusively in nails injured by shoes that are too small or ill-fitted, causing pressure damage to the tissue under the end of the nail.[27] This tissue then retracts and allows the fungus to penetrate the vulnerable undersurface of the nail plate. The pity is that it is incredibly difficult to buy women's shoes that fit properly. They are almost all made on European or Oriental lasts designed for the average foot of those locations. Unfortunately the average American foot is shaped differently (bigger, for one thing).

Hair

Hair, like the skin's stratum corneum, is mostly a nonliving keratin protein. The hair shaft is located deep in the dermis. The root, at the base of the hair follicle, is the only living and growing part of the hair. Each hair is made up of two parts, the cortex and the cuticle. The cortex is the center support layer, and the cuticle is the outer protective layer. The hair grows in three cycles: the growing (anagen) phase, the resting (telogen) phase, and the falling-out (catagen) phase. Approximately 85 percent of the time is spent in the growing phase, 11 percent in the resting phase, and the remaining 4 percent in the falling-out phase. A woman has an average of approximately 125,000 strands of hair on her head and loses between 50 to 100 hairs a day. There is more hair loss in the late fall, less hair loss in the spring. When a hair falls out, the same hair follicle is used to grow a new hair. Actually, when a hair falls out under normal circumstances, it does so because it is being pushed out by a newly growing replacement hair. Generally, scalp hair grows about one-half to three-fourths inch a month. Genetic factors determine hair type, quantity, pattern, and location.

Hair and Aging

During middle age, most women's hair thins and turns gray or white. The good news is that few women really lose all their hair. Generally, thinning is most prominent at the crown, and hair also becomes thinner and finer in the temporal area. Again, the amount of the loss is usually dependent on heredity. However, health factors, such as stress and illness and reactions to certain drugs, notably beta-blockers, can cause hair loss. Currently the only approved medical treatment for common female hair loss with aging is Rogaine,[28] now available over-the-counter. Finasteride (Propecia[29]), another drug to prevent hair loss, has recently been released, but because of hormonal effects is only used in men.

Also, with aging, the pigment cells disappear from the hair follicle. The number of the melanocytes begins to diminish at about the age of 30. Gray hair is the result of only a few melanocytes in the hair follicle and white hair results from an absence of melanocytes. Gray hair is very strong and more resistant to permanents and dyes. Gray hair tends to have thicker strands and can look beautiful and full.

Hirsutism

When the estrogen level drops and becomes erratic, the balance between estrogen and androgen is disrupted. This may cause hirsutism—the growth of new, thick, coarse, dark hairs appearing usually in unwanted areas of the body. Also, a couple of medical disorders can cause the problem, so if more than a few "wild hairs" appear, it might be best to consult a physician.

Vaginal and Urinary Tracts

The vagina is a very adaptable part of the body. It can elongate, stretch, and lubricate itself for sexual activity. It also has the ability to accommodate the birth of a child and return to its original shape.

In early adulthood the vagina is quite acidic, which helps prevent infection. As women age and approach menopause, less estrogen is produced, causing a decrease in production of vaginal fluids and an alkaline shift in the vaginal pH. The vaginal entrance becomes smaller, the vaginal epidermis becomes thinner and less elastic, and the self-lubricating ability of the vagina diminishes. These changes may result in more frequent vaginal infections and discomfort or pain during sexual intercourse.

Also, the bladder and the urethra over time begin to lose muscle tone. These physical changes in the urethra, bladder, and vagina can leave the urethra more exposed to trauma from sexual activity. Combined with a reduction of fluids, these changes increase the risk of bladder infection and inflammation. Incontinence is another common problem associated with the loss of muscle tone. Loss of urinary control can be trivial to extreme. Often this problem is exacerbated by the onset of menopause and drop in estrogen. Kegel exercises have been used successfully for years to improve bladder control. (See Chapter 26.) Medications are also used to relieve the problem.

Vaginitis actually comprises a number of disorders, but they all cause an inflammation of the vagina with burning, itching, soreness, and a sometimes odorous discharge. Different factors contribute to vaginitis: antibiotics, douches, deodorants, nylon underwear and pantyhose, wet bathing suits, bath oils and bubble baths, tight pants, intercourse with inadequate lubrication, and intercourse with an infected partner.

As women age, some have more difficulties than others. Some experience little discomfort while others are miserable. However, most women encounter problems to some degree or another. Hopefully they will talk to their physicians about solutions, especially when some of the more embarrassing problems, such as incontinence, occur. Always see a physician if problems persist. Many infections and physical discomforts may be signs of other more serious problems.

You are not alone. After all, this is the generation of the baby boomers. It has been estimated that close to 19 million women next year alone will enter menopause.

Miscellaneous Skin Nutrients and Treatments

Vitamin C

Some dermatologists recommend vitamin C to promote healthy skin. Quite a bit of evidence exists that C speeds up wound healing. (See Chapter 5.)

Vitamin E

Along with vitamin C, vitamin E is a major antioxidant and preventer of inflammation and tissue injury.

Vitamin A

Vitamin A is associated with the development of healthy mucous membranes. (See Chapter 3.)

Aloe Vera

There is some evidence that aloe vera can help alleviate radiation dermatitis. It also promotes healing in chronic leg ulcers, pressure sores, frostbite, and surgical wounds. Unfortunately, few controlled studies have been done with humans.[30, 31]

Biotin

Biotin promotes healthy hair and skin. (See Chapter 4.)

Calcium

The skin has a calcium-dependent antioxidant enzyme. It has been suggested that a calcium deficiency can accelerate skin aging. (See Chapter 11.)

Copper

Copper is involved with the production of elastin, collagen, and melanin. (See Chapter 13.)

Zinc

Zinc has been reported to increase the speed of wound and ulcer healing. (See Chapter 22.)

Retin-A

This popular drug has been shown to improve photo-aged skin.[32, 33] Researchers are not actually sure why the medication works. However, improvements have been noted in fine wrinkling, elasticity, and skin color.

Laser Resurfacing for the Treatment of Facial Wrinkles and Scars

Susan S. Roper, M.D.

Carbon dioxide laser resurfacing today provides a highly accurate method of resurfacing and rejuvenating the skin. Laser resurfacing of the skin initially developed in the 1980s with the continuous wave CO_2 lasers in a defocused mode to vaporize the skin's surface, used primarily to treat a precancerous condition of the lips known as actinic cheilitis.[34, 35, 36] These initial resurfacing lasers, however, lacked the precision to resurface the skin predictably for cosmetic use. Two laser systems for cosmetic use were ultimately develeoped in the late 1980s and early 1990s that could remove the desired amount of tissue without damaging the surrounding skin with nonspecific heat conduction: the Ultrapulse[37] system and the Sharplan Silktouch[38] flashscanner system.[39, 40, 41, 42, 43, 44, 45, 46, 47, 48, 49, 50] Most of the research on CO_2 laser resurfacing has come from studying these two systems; however, other systems in the past few years have been developed using similar technology. Many physicians saw the advantages of resurfacing with a laser over previous resurfacing techniques using chemical peels or dermabrasion. These advantages include precise control of resurfacing depth, surface contouring, immediate visual assessment of wrinkle removal, lack of bleeding, and less postoperative pain and swelling.[51]

Carbon dioxide lasers emit light at 10,600 nanometers (nm), which is absorbed by water in the skin. This laser-tissue interaction heats the water in the skin and is capable of precisely removing a tenth of a millimeter (mm) of the skin's surface without significant thermal damage to surrounding tissue. To do this requires a laser with pulse duration of less than 1 millisecond (ms), such as the Coherent Ultrapulse or Sharplan Silktouch systems. The energy of the laser has to be sufficient so that the surface of the skin is not "cooked" but vaporized cleanly. When the skin is vaporized in such a manner, the zone of thermal damage with one pass of the laser measures only 1/20 to 1/10 mm. Removal of surface irregularities with optimal skin healing occurs. To remove deep wrinkles, however, often more than one pass of the laser is necessary. With each pass, the zone of residual thermal damage increases, resulting in contraction and tightening of the skin.[52] The skin thickness on the face varies from 0.5 mm in the eyelid area to 2.0 mm on the cheeks. The laser surgeon tailors the number of laser passes at each site depending on the location and depth of the wrinkles. Upon healing, the wrinkles are significantly improved. Results can be enhanced with subsequent treatments, if desired.

Indications for laser resurfacing include treatment of facial wrinkles, sun-damaged skin, acne scarring, and scarring from surgery or previous accidents. When the Coherent Ultrapulse and Sharplan Silktouch resurfacing lasers were first developed, the skin around the lips became the most popular area for resurfacing. This traditionally was the most difficult area to resurface with any technology, and the advent of the laser to precisely remove these lip lines was hailed as miraculous. Then it was discovered that the laser not only smoothed these lip lines, but tightened the skin around them as well. This led to more full-face laser resurfacing procedures, where the skin tightens and acquires the appearance of face-lift. The majority of the tightening of the skin is seen by 6 months after the procedure; however, the skin's surface improves for 12 months and longer after the procedure. Research has shown that not only new collagen formation improves the laser-resurfaced skin, but new elastic fiber formation as well.[53] The laser removes the sun damage in the surface of the skin that causes aging and may also decrease the incidence of skin cancer in these areas. It smooths the skin and retexturizes it. The pores may appear less noticeable. Acne scars and surgery scars are diminished by 25 to 50 percent. Results are reported to be excellent for mild acne scarring and moderate for severe acne scarring. Patients with severe, deep acne scarring may require adjunctive procedures for best results.[54, 55]

Since the laser resurfacing procedure requires re-epithelialization of the skin, one must usually allow 7 to 14 days for initial healing. The more passes the laser surgeon takes to remove the wrinkles, the longer it takes to heal, and the longer the postlaser erythema (redness). This can be camouflaged easily afterward with certain waterproof camouflage makeup systems. The laser surgeon should provide advice and help in this area. Most of the erythema is resolved by three to six months. There does exists patient-to-patient variability on length of time to heal. Certain environmental factors will delay healing, such as cigarette smoking.[56] Most laser surgeons ask their patients to decrease their cigarette smoking while healing, or to quit smoking before the procedure. It is important that the skin not be allowed to dry out significantly in the healing process, as this will delay healing time. Each laser surgeon has developed a postlaser healing plan to minimize healing time. Some surgeons prefer a closed-bandage system, and some prefer a more open system. Some use a combination of the two. One study showed that the quickest healing system used a hydrogel bandage such as Vigilon[57] or 2nd Skin.[58, 59] All surgeons put their patients on medication to prevent herpes simplex during the healing process and use antibacterial regimes to prevent infection.[60, 61] Some laser surgeons also recommend that patients undergoing face-lift procedures not be simultaneously resurfaced since impaired blood supply may cause abnormal healing.[62] This may not be a problem if only the perioral area is resurfaced.

Laser surgeons differ in their recommendations for pretreatment of the skin prior to laser resurfacing. Some laser surgeons find that pretreatment of the skin with retinoic acid or alpha-hydroxy acids speed healing,[63] whereas others do not find them to hasten the healing process at all.[64, 65] Some recommend that patients with moderately tanning skin and darker be pretreated with hydroquinone to decrease the incidence of postlaser hyperpigmentation (darkening). Most laser surgeons agree on posttreating the skin with retinoic acid, azelaic acid, or glycolic acid after healing is complete. The use of topical hydroquinone for darker skin types is recommended by most laser surgeons in the posttreatment period to prevent temporary hyperpigmentation, which is most common in the first three months after laser resurfacing.[66, 67]

Posttreatment erythema is an expected aftereffect of CO_2 laser resurfacing, and usually resolves by three to six months after treatment, depending on the depth of the resurfacing procedure and the skin type of the patient. This posttreatment erythema is linked to the thermal effect on collagen from the CO_2 laser.[68, 69, 70] Some of this thermal effect, however, is thought to be necessary to achieve one of the desired laser effects on the skin: the tightening that is seen in the healing process.[71, 72] The Erbium:yag resurfacing laser was developed to avoid posttreatment erythma and speed healing times. The Erbium:yag laser removes 1/100 to 4/100 mm of the surface of the skin with each laser pass, compared to 1/10 of a mm with the CO_2 laser. Quicker healing is observed after the Erbium laser, and postoperative erythema resolves in less than two weeks.[73, 74] More passes are needed to remove deeper wrinkles, however; and experienced laser surgeons find the deeper wrinkles more easily removed with the CO_2 laser than with the Erbium laser. Sharplan Silktouch added a Feathertouch[75] unit to their laser system to be used in areas where more superficial laser resurfacing is desired, giving healing times and decreased erythema similar to the Erbium:yag laser. The Tru-Pulse[76] CO_2 laser also claims enhanced healing and minimized posttreatment erythema.[77]

Another occasional side effect of laser resurfacing that can be seen afterward is exacerbation of acne and perioral dermatitis.[78] Occasionally a tendency to rosacea can be aggravated, which is best treated with oral antibiotics. Since allergies to topical preparations are common following laser resurfacing, bland emollients are easier for patients to tolerate in the posttreatment period. Posttreatment hyperpigmentation in the first three months can frequently occur, especially in darker skin types, but is easily controlled or prevented using a combination of azelaic acid, glycolic acid, retinoic acid, and/or hydroquinone. Delayed hypopigmentation has been seen in some patients after 6 to 12 months.

More severe complications include infection, herpes simplex infection being the most serious. For this reason, all patients are now pretreated with an antiviral medication for herpes prior to laser resurfacing and kept on it until healed. Bacterial and yeast infection can also occur, which are usually preventable. Other severe complications include abnormal scarring, allergic reactions to anesthesia, inadvertant eye injury, and ectropion (abnormal healing of the eyelids). The risk of abnormal scarring increases immediately after isotretinoin (Accutane[79]) use. All Accutane patients are advised to wait 12 to 24 months after finishing Accutane before having laser resurfacing. A history of prior cosmetic procedures and a tendency to form keloids may be risk factors for abnormal healing after laser resurfacing.

Any laser system can potentially result in scarring and tissue damage; therefore, adequate education and skill in the laser surgeon are essential when utilizing the resurfacing lasers. The distinct advantages of the laser resurfacing systems as a precise method of removal of wrinkles, sun damage, and scars are enormous, and many patients are seeking skilled physicians performing laser resurfacing to improve their appearance. Laser resurfacing is quickly replacing dermabrasion and chemical peels in popularity, yielding results that many see as superior and providing a means of rejuvenation in patients who are not otherwise surgical candidates.

34

Weight

As PREVIOUSLY mentioned, lean body mass or muscle mass decreases as we age. The percentage of fat goes up, and the amount of muscle goes down. Every year from our middle 30s on, the body requires fewer and fewer calories per day to maintain the same weight. The number of calories necessary to maintain weight declines by an estimated 2 to 8 percent per decade.[1]

Ideal body weight is not what is glamorized by the media or preferred by couturiers. It is a matter of health, not fashion; and it can easily be computed or looked up in appropriate charts. (See Height and Weight Table in this chapter.) Women who are 15 percent below the average weight have higher risks of pneumonia, influenza (the *real* flu), digestive-system disorders, ischemic heart disease, and death.[2] This may be due to decreased energy intake rather than low weight per se.[3] Obese women (30 percent or more over ideal body weight)[4] increase their risk of diabetes, high blood pressure, and death.[5,6]

The relationship between weight and mortality can be viewed as a U-shaped curve. The top of one end of the curve represents the very heavy people and the top of the other end represents the very thin people. Both of these extremes have high mortality rates. This pattern has also been found to be true for the hospitalization rate.[7] One 12-year study comparing mortality and body weight reviewed more than 17,000 healthy, nonsmoking Finnish women between ages 25 and 79.

Researchers found that thin and obese women between ages 25 and 64 had the highest mortality. However, this pattern of mortality did not hold for women over 64.[8]

Many studies show that the above-mentioned mortality and body weight curves may be true for middle-aged people but not for older people. Older people appear to require more weight for a given height than younger people. People 60 and older tend to have a higher mortality associated with thinness than those under that age.[9]

There is lower mortality among obese people who maintain their weight than among those whose weights fluctuate. A modest, 10 percent or less, weight reduction over an 18-month period should be the desired goal. After that goal has been achieved another reduction can be considered. This modest reduction also appears to have the greatest overall health benefits.[10] One study on weight gain and cardiovascular health followed almost 12,000 Harvard alumni with a mean age of 58 over a 10-year period. Originally, the men were free of cardiovascular disease. Based on the men's questionnaires, the study concluded that significant body weight *gain or loss* was associated with a higher rate of mortality from coronary heart disease and other noncancer causes.[11] Intentional weight loss by overweight, white, U.S. women consistently reduced mortality in those with obesity-related illness. Modest intentional weight loss is associated with increased longevity in individuals.[12]

Ideal Body Weight

A recent survey found that about 40 percent of adult women are trying to lose weight at any one time. The bad news is that it hardly ever works.[13] Be careful of yo-yo dieting; cyclically losing and regaining weight may be detrimental to overall health. When an individual loses 20 pounds quickly, that weight loss represents 5 pounds of muscle and 15 pounds of fat. With resumption of a normal diet, the body, now adjusted to starvation metabolism, has lower caloric needs. Now the body requires fewer calories to maintain weight, and when the 20 pounds are regained, 18 pounds are fat and 2 pounds are muscle.[14] And to top it off, the weight lost is usually back within two years. Significant reductions in total bone mineral density have been found in obese women who consumed very low-calorie diets of 925 calories per day. Also, diet plus resistance training was not associated with a significantly better outcome. These findings raise concerns because of the incredible popularity of dieting among American women.[15]

See the following Height and Weight Table for women aged 25 to 59 based on the lowest mortality. The weight is measured in pounds according to frame size, including 3 pounds of clothing and 1-inch heels.

Height and Weight Table for Women Aged 25 to 59

Height in Feet and Inches	Small Frame	Medium Frame	Large Frame
4′10″	102–111	109–121	118–131
4′11″	103–113	111–123	120–134
5′0″	104–115	113–126	122–137
5′1″	106–118	115–129	125–140
5′2″	108–121	118–132	128–143
5′3″	111–124	121–135	131–147
5′4″	114–127	124–138	134–151
5′5″	117–130	127–141	137–155
5′6″	120–133	130–144	140–159
5′7″	123–136	133–147	143–163
5′8″	126–139	136–150	146–167
5′9″	129–142	139–153	149–170
5′10″	132–145	142–156	152–173
5′11″	135–148	145–159	155–176
6′0″	138–151	148–162	158–179

Reprinted courtesy of Metropolitan Life Insurance Company.

Another way to check your weight is by the body mass index (BMI). BMI is calculated by dividing your weight in kilograms by height in meters squared. Or look at the following chart. A BMI of 19 to 25 is OK, 26 or 27 is high, and over 27 is very high.[16] For more information, con-

Body Mass Index Chart (BMI)

Body Weight (pounds)

Height (inches)	19	20	21	22	23	24	25	26	27	28	29	30	31	32	33	34	35	36	37
58	91	96	100	105	110	115	119	124	129	134	138	143	148	153	158	162	167	172	177
59	94	99	104	109	114	119	124	128	133	138	143	148	153	158	163	168	173	178	183
60	97	102	107	112	118	123	128	133	138	143	148	153	158	163	168	174	179	184	189
61	100	106	111	116	122	127	132	137	143	148	153	158	164	169	174	180	185	190	195
62	104	109	115	120	126	131	136	142	147	153	158	164	169	175	180	186	191	196	202
63	107	113	118	124	130	135	141	146	152	158	163	169	175	180	186	191	197	203	208
64	110	116	122	128	134	140	145	151	157	163	169	174	180	186	192	197	204	209	215
65	114	120	126	132	138	144	150	156	162	168	174	180	186	192	198	204	210	216	222
66	118	124	130	136	142	148	155	161	167	173	179	186	192	198	204	210	216	223	229
67	121	127	134	140	146	153	159	166	172	178	185	191	198	204	211	217	223	230	236

Height (inches)	38	39	40	41	42	43	44	45	46	47	48	49	50	51	52	53	54
58	181	186	191	196	201	205	210	215	220	224	229	234	239	244	248	253	258
59	188	193	198	203	208	212	217	222	227	232	237	242	247	252	257	262	267
60	194	199	204	209	215	220	225	230	235	240	245	250	255	261	266	271	276
61	201	206	211	217	222	227	232	238	243	248	254	259	264	269	275	280	285
62	207	213	218	224	229	235	240	246	251	256	262	267	273	278	284	289	295
63	214	220	225	231	237	242	248	254	259	265	270	278	282	287	293	299	304
64	221	227	232	238	244	250	256	262	267	273	279	285	291	296	302	308	314
65	228	234	240	246	252	258	264	270	276	282	288	294	300	306	312	318	324
66	235	241	247	253	260	266	272	278	284	291	297	303	309	315	322	328	334
67	242	249	255	261	268	274	280	287	293	299	306	312	319	325	331	338	344

sult the website of the National Heart, Lung, and Blood Institute, www.nhlbi.nih.gov.

To use this table, find the appropriate height in the left-hand column. Move across to a given weight. The number at the top of the column is the BMI at that height and weight. Pounds have been rounded off.

Losing Weight

Weight reduction is a $30 billion industry in this country. Diet books year after year rank number one in book sales.[17] Drug companies and supplemental pill manufacturers dream and scheme of marketing the "new diet" fix. However, even with all the marketing, no evidence exists that there has been a lasting decrease in obesity. Be careful. Recently many weight-reducing drugs that worked have disappeared because of dangerous side effects. And unfortunately most of that weight that was lost is back.

Ephedrine is a commonly used diet aid. An ephedrine/caffeine combination has been shown to be effective in maintaining weight loss while preserving lean body mass. Some researchers claim that the side effects are minor and transient and that there are no withdrawal symptoms.[18] However, other reports have blamed chronic ephedrine use for causing delusional disorders as well as manic conditions.[19] The drug may also predispose people to strokes.[20]

Chromium picolinate is another dietary supplement that has gained popularity for weight reduction. It has been noted that picolinic acid affects the metabolism of serotonin, dopamine, and norepinephrine in the brain. Individuals with behavior disorders should be wary of the supplements. It may exaggerate schizophrenia and can cause psychotic behaviors.[21] In a study including active Navy personnel, 79 men and 16 women, chromium picolinate was ineffective in aiding fat reduction. It was not recommended to be a part of the Navy weight loss programs.[22]

Pantothenic acid may be a significant help to dieters. During aggressive dieting, the metabolism of body fat is incomplete, resulting in the production of waste products, creating hunger, weakness, and ketosis. With the addition of pantothenic acid, the ketosis may be circumvented. As a result, a sufficient amount of energy would be released from storage fat to relieve dieters of the sense of hunger and weakness that otherwise would be difficult to endure. It is thought that maintaining an ample supply of pantothenic acid in the body allows the efficient conversion of fat to energy. To maintain weight, 1 to 3 g of pantothenic acid together with a careful diet was needed; 2.5 g of pantothenic acid was given to patients during aggressive dieting (1,000 cal per day). No side effects have been observed in patients at 10 grams a day.[23]

Common sense, although we sometimes don't want to hear it, makes sense. To lose weight, you need to reduce calories and increase exercise. Caloric intake required for weight maintenance can be calculated simply. An active person should multiply her present weight in pounds by 15 (calories). A not-so-active person should multiply her weight by 13 (calories). This will give the total number of calories per day needed to maintain weight. For most women, losing 1 or 2 pounds of weight per week requires reducing daily calories to 1,200 to 1,500.[24] Remember, a pound is worth 3,500 calories. Losing and maintaining weight requires a change in attitude and food choices forever.

Part IV

Alternative Therapies

Today patients need to be good consumers. Understanding the nature of the different primary health care providers is essential in order to choose the options available. The following articles on acupuncture, chiropractic, and osteopathy and allopathy are written by specialists in their fields of medicine and describe some of the similarities and differences. Each has its role in the world of health care.

35

Acupuncture, Herbs, and Traditional Chinese Medicine

Mary Felicia Bochichio, A.P., D.A., Dipl. Ac.

ACUPUNCTURE HAS become very popular over the past few years. What most Americans need to understand is that it is actually only one form of treatment utilized in the ancient medical practice of *traditional Chinese medicine* (TCM). TCM is the fundamental cornerstone and basis for the practice of acupuncture, Chinese herbology and tui na (Chinese massage and bodywork). This full system of medicine, along with its ancient diagnostic techniques, has an impressive history that dates back more than 2,500 years. It comes as no surprise that the use of Chinese herbs and acupuncture has gained such an enormous amount of media exposure over the past few years.

The National Institute of Health, (NIH), World Health Organization (WHO), and the Food and Drug Administration (FDA) have all given their stamp of approval on various aspects of the ancient practice of acupuncture. *Life* magazine featured two cover stories, "The Healing Revolution" and "The Healing Power of Touch," within a 12-month period of time. *Time* magazine, *U.S. News and World Report*, and *Newsweek* as well as the *New York Times*, *Miami Herald*, and the *Wall Street Journal* have all featured articles about America's fascination and trend toward embracing this ancient medical art.

With the increase in media and government attention, a significant increase in public demand has occurred. A large portion of this demand is coming from American women. They want to educate themselves about preventive health care to keep themselves and their families healthy. They are searching for safer and more cost-effective methods and treatments for many of the diseases that they or their families suffer from. American women have been eagerly waiting to hear about the many benefits of this ancient medical art that utilizes acupuncture, Chinese herbs, and other natural remedies. They recognize the benefits of the safe, ancient practice referred to as TCM.

TCM directly balances energy levels in the body similar to the way Western medical science balances the chemistry in the body. Both Eastern and Western medical science agree that balance, or homeostasis, is necessary to achieve optimum health. TCM directly balances energy levels to achieve optimum health.

The idea of balance is not new. In fact, the first time someone thought of the idea of balance was probably close to 5,000 years ago in the Eastern Himalayas. Balance is what all the forces of nature strive for; it is the most basic force of life. It is a basic concept in physics, mathematics, electronics, mechanics, and many other modern disciplines. Life can survive on this planet because there is a delicate environmental balance. This entire physical universe exists and continues because it is in balance.

Western science caught up with the idea of balance some time around Galileo's time. The resulting evolution of the investigation into natural balance tracks Newton's work on gravity and inertia (for every action there is an equal and opposite reaction) and Einstein's theory of relativity, $E=Mc^2$ (the exact definition of the balance between mass and energy that defines time as the measurement of change). Western scientists have been working on the application of balance for a few hundred years, but all they can actually do with it is parlor tricks like thermonuclear explosions. Eastern science, or Eastern philosophy, has been investigating balance for thousands of years and can produce truly useful results such as effectively treating a headache.

Why this difference of application of balance? Let's take a quick look at history. Both science and religion agree that life started in the general area of the Mesopotamia River Valley. We generally consider everything west of this point to be "Western" and everything east of it to be "Eastern." It is generally agreed that after man began his first society it expanded in two directions—East and West. To the West lay lush forests, game, farmland, and plentiful resources. The environment was not that challenging. Solutions to the problems of survival were most often solved immediately with direct application of force, even at the expense of the resources. To the East lay vast regions with very scarce resources. The problems of survival were solved through perseverance and economy of resources.

The medical technology developed in the East is based on preserving and balancing the resources or the forces of the body. Underlying Eastern medicine is the philosophy of yin and yang. Yin and yang are the two primary forces in balance in the universe. Men are yang and women are yin, day is yang and night is yin. There is a natural balance of yin and yang, and when it is forced out of balance, systems are stressed and may stop functioning. For example, when there is too much stress (yang), relaxation (yin) becomes necessary and if not reconciled, physiological systems go out of balance and illness results.

Western medical technology was developed to address acute conditions immediately, such as patching up a hole from a sword or repairing a broken leg—quick, immediate direct application of force to eliminate symptoms. Eastern medical technology took a more chronic approach and was much more effective with illness until Western technology advanced to the point that the "cure by force" philosophy could be directly applied to bacteria. But look what's happening now—the staphylococcus bacteria has become resistant to every antibiotic except one, and in Japan it recently showed signs of resistance to that one. Nature is balancing the scale again.

In this philosophy of balance, the balance is not static. It flows one way and then the other. The very symbol for yin and yang shows these surges in balance and implies a cycle. This philosophy postulates that the most basic manifestation of nature, or the most basic manifestation of life, is that energy generated by living things is enhanced by the achievement of balance. Now remember, this is not a static state of balance or equilibrium; it is more like a pendulum, or a sine wave for the more technically minded. The balance is achieved over time by leaning first one way and then the other. In this state the force becomes stronger. It's like playing on a swing. You apply force one way, then the other; and you swing higher and higher. When the energy is balanced there is more energy generated. When it's imbalanced, it's like trying to just swing frontward without ever going backward. It's hard to build up any energy.

In Eastern medicine, or more specifically traditional Chinese medicine (TCM), there is a defined balance of forces in the body. When these forces are in balance, you are healthy and unlikely to succumb to a disease. Not impossible by any means, because another strong influence may stress you enough to cause you to use your own forces in such a way as to cause an imbalance, making you again susceptible to disease.

Western medicine is a manifestation of the Western philosophy of direct application of force. "Kill the germ directly with a direct application of force" with an antibiotic, a laser, chemotherapy, or a scalpel. Eastern medicine is an application of the Eastern philosophy of preserving and balancing the resources. "Balance the forces in the body and the body will deal with the germ." Now both of these philosophies and the resulting medical technology borrow a great deal from one another, but for the most part they are distinctly different. They both have their strong points and weak points and are in general very complementary.

Western medical technology is very effective when properly applied in the correct circumstance. Eastern medicine is also very effective when properly applied in the correct circumstance. The trick is in the balance. It seems, however, that most Western societies have become stuck in the rut of trying to use one solution for every problem.

While physical rehabilitation and holistic care have become popular recently, Western medicine essentially has had three traditional answers for illness: drugs, surgery, or live with it. Kill it with drugs, cut it out with a scalpel, or live with the problem. While Western medical technology has always been effective for injuries, it did very poorly with illness until the discovery of the antibiotic and vaccine. This allowed the philosophy of force to be applied at a cellular level.

Western medical technology has been more effective for injuries and acute conditions, and Eastern medical technology has always been more effective with health maintenance and prevention.

Injuries are caused by external force; the impact of the body forcefully contacting a foreign object such as a fall or a punch in the nose. Illness is caused by an imbalance of internal forces, such as too many germs and not enough white cells, or too much work and not enough rest, or too much yin and not enough yang.

Many people still believe that not having any acute symptoms means you are healthy. A Western physician may even have told them that. Many believe that you can be tired all the time, have poor digestion, backaches, or headaches, and still be "healthy."

If you watch TV, you may have noticed that every other ad you see promotes an over-the-counter drug for some "normal" problem. It must be normal to have headaches all the time; look at how much Tylenol is sold. Well, it is not "normal" to have headaches, it is just common. A cold is not normal, it is common. Normal would imply that it's supposed to be there; it is not.

Eastern medical philosophy tells us that for any of these symptoms to be occurring, you are already out of balance and susceptible to disease. Masking symptoms with drugs does not restore the balance.

All of us have experienced being around germs and not getting sick. The germs we inhale put stress on our system. The body has to manufacture antibodies to handle those germs and that uses up resources and creates an imbalance of forces in the body. Now in most cases your body can fully restore its own balance. When you're short on energy, you sleep and get back in balance. But what if you don't? What if you're tired and have been under stress? An imbalance at work, home, in the body—they all stress nature's drive for balance. You would be more likely to get sick from those germs if you were under stress.

It has been well established that stress predisposes you to getting sick. Stress is caused by an imbalance. According to TCM, when energy levels in your body are imbalanced, you are much more likely to get sick. When you are sick, the forces in your body are definitely out of balance.

For thousands of years, many of the East's greatest minds have worked to understand the natural balance of energy levels in the human body. Through those thousands of years of effort, experimentation, trial and error, these great minds have achieved a great deal of success in identifying the various forces in the body and how they interact. We have identified these forces and can directly manipulate them to some degree to restore their balance. (I say "we have identified" because I consider myself a part of this tradition and invite you to feel the same way. When I say "Eastern" or "Western," I am only talking about origins. All knowledge belongs to mankind.)

TCM's Integration with Western Medicine

Western science is based on the identification of laws, the operation of which can be reliably demonstrated through experimentation. In order for science to consider something "true," it has to be able to predict an experimental result with a high degree of accuracy. A basic law of electronics is Ohms Law, which defines the exact predictable balance between current, voltage, and resistance in an electrical circuit. These changes can be exactly reproduced by any experimenter anywhere in the world, so Western science says it is true. The same principal applies to Pasture's experiment, and it applies to the exact predictable results of the introduction of penicillin into a culture of the E. Coli bacteria. These are accepted principles because they produce reliable, predictable results under experimentation.

From a Western perspective, there are far more "unknowns" than "knowns" in medicine. Eastern medical philosophy is based on balancing the energy levels or electronics of the body. Science knows next to nothing about the electronics of the body. We can only take some very gross measurements because we don't have the technology to really measure the energy fields in and around the body. They are just too small. We can stick a needle into a nerve or muscle and measure the voltage, but we can't compare the characteristics of the field around the right arm to the characteristics of the field around the left arm; however, we can prove mathematically that they are there. We can get an image of something with Kirilian photography, but we don't really know what it means.

We know those fields are there because we know a little something about energy. We know that anytime a current moves through a conductor it creates a field. We also know that if we create a field around a conductor, a current will flow. This gives us motors and generators. Every time an electrical charge moves along a nerve it is creating a field. That field is also being affected by the fields generated by other charges moving along other nerves. Hopefully, those fields will all be in resonance (or balance) and reinforce each other.

It just so happens that sticking an antenna (or acupuncture needle) into the body in the right place can allow the energy levels to resonate, or come into balance or harmony. You just have to know how the energy levels flow and where to "stick" the antenna.

It is plain to see that these fields can be very important but they cannot be measured with today's technology. We can measure the stronger fields created by the brain and large nerves with devices such as the EEG, EMG, and EKG, but these are the exception rather than the rule. Trying to measure such a small field is like trying to hear someone whisper on the other side of a football stadium in the final two minutes of a game. There is so much electrical energy in our environment today that it makes measuring these fields impossible. Look around at all the wires in your life. We are exposed to millions of times more electrical energy fields than our grandparents.

It is interesting that without as much as an ohmmeter or a cyclotron, the ancient developers of TCM mapped the patterns of energy in the body and developed the means to manipulate them to restore the balance in the body. They did this through 2,500 years of research, experimentation, and development. Over the course of time, the energy fields were identified along with their interactions with the various physiological systems of the body through trial and error and observation. Utilizing thousands of years of documentation, practitioners have learned how to affect this energy to restore balance in the body.

Documented physiological effects of acupuncture include a release of endorphins (the body's natural painkiller) and an increase in blood circulation. This is why it is so effective for pain-related conditions, both acute and chronic. Acupuncture can aid in the treatment of injuries to reduce the amount of pain medications that are needed and enhance the healing process. Many athletes are discovering that this is a great benefit, considering the side effects of many of the drug treatments, such as steroids, that are commonly used.

It is important to understand and remember that the effects of acupuncture and herbs have a cumulative effect. When first undergoing care, it is necessary to receive treatments more often to build the effects. As they build, the effects last longer. A course of treatment for acupuncture can be from 8 to 15 treatments. With some chronic conditions, a patient may not respond until the sixth treatment. With some acute conditions, a patient's response can be very quick with only a few treatments needed. A course of treatment with herbs can be as short as a few days or last up to several months. It really depends on the individual patient, the condition, and the amount of time the problem has existed. A comprehensive evaluation of the patient will enable the practitioner to outline a treatment protocol and discuss the patient's expectations and responsibilities.

Herbology and TCM

Chinese herbology, acupuncture, and tui na (massage) are the three main treatment modalities used by TCM practitioners for restoring balance in the body. Herbal recommendations along with acupuncture treatments are a common protocol for many conditions. Herbal therapy plays a vital role in the treatment of chronic, internal diseases that have weakened the body's systems.

There is a general public opinion that just because something is natural, it is safe. This is not true about Chinese herbology. The practice of Chinese herbology uses both single herbs as well as herbal formulas containing several herbs. Ancient texts document various herbal formulas that can be used to treat various conditions. When herbs are combined, there is a synergistic effect that results in precise effective treatment. TCM developed the practice of herbology to coincide with treating the energy (Qi) imbalance in the body. Ancient texts categorize the herbs according to their properties, channel entered, organs affected, taste, temperature, toxicity, and disease or symptom. A disease can only be treated after the imbalance in the energy levels (Qi) of the body has been identified.

The oldest known significant Chinese medical text, *Yellow Emperor's Inner Classic* (Huang Di Nei Jing), was compiled between 200 B.C. and 100 B.C. This ancient text outlines the theoretical and philosophical foundation of TCM. With an understanding of this foundation, a practitioner can diagnose the imbalance and then incorporate herbs and acupuncture into a treatment protocol.

A disease classified by Western medicine, such as sinusitis, can actually be broken down into many different types or imbalances, according to TCM. This is probably why some people respond to certain drugs for this condition and others do not. Premenstrual syndrome (PMS) can be differentiated according to TCM diagnostics into at least five different categories. Therefore, the treatment protocol and herbal recommendations depend on the proper TCM diagnosis of the imbalance. Herbal prescriptions are not based on just a symptom or disease. In fact, a condition could worsen if the wrong herb or formula is recommended. So remember, just because it worked for someone else with the same disease or symptom does not mean that it is appropriate for you. The patient must be diagnosed according to TCM diagnostic techniques before herbal recommendations can be made. Another example is asthma, which can be broken down into several different types according to TCM. So just because a particular herb or herbal formula worked well for your neighbor's asthma, does not mean it will have the same effect for you. In fact, it could even make you worse if your imbalance is the opposite of your neighbor's. For any disease, it is recommended that you seek the advice of a qualified, licensed TCM practitioner before experimenting with herbs for the treatment of disease.

TCM as a Form of Primary Health Care

What makes TCM so unique is that it is a full medical system that utilizes ancient diagnostic techniques to determine a patient's imbalance in her energy levels, or Qi as the ancient texts refer to it. We look at the individual as a whole, not just a particular problem or disease. Using the diagnostic techniques developed by TCM, we can identify the imbalance and treat it accordingly. Once the body's systems are stimulated to return to balance, symptoms diminish or disappear. TCM views disease as an imbalance. Once the imbalance is treated, the body takes care of the rest. With more complex disease conditions where the body is severely weakened, the quality of life can be enhanced with treatment. Once the patient is properly diagnosed and the treatment principle is determined, the practitioner can then develop a treatment protocol. This can include acupuncture, herbs, tui na (Chinese massage), moxibustion (heat), cupping, or the modern techniques of magnetic, electric, and laser acupuncture.

Many refer to this ancient medical art as "alternative" health care. Doesn't it make more sense that the "alternative" be the drastic approach and the "primary" be the safer, noninvasive, cost-efficient approach that TCM offers? As this ancient art integrates into America's health care system, many will agree that benefits of such integration will aid in enhancing the overall health of our entire nation. Some of the many conditions that can be helped by TCM include the following.

Gynecological:

- PMS, cramps, pain
- Irregular periods
- Menopause
- Morning sickness

Respiratory:

- Colds and flu
- Bronchitis
- Sinusitis
- Asthma
- Allergies
- Chronic cough
- Digestive
- Ulcers
- Colitis
- Indigestion
- Diarrhea
- Constipation

Eyes, Ears, Nose, Throat, Dental:

- Earaches
- Poor eyesight
- Rhinitis
- Tonsillitis
- Sore throat, laryngitis

- TMJ
- Postextraction pain
- Muscular, skeletal

Neurologic:

- Headache
- Migraine
- Arthritis
- Neuralgia
- Sciatica
- Back pain
- Muscle spasm
- Bursitis
- Tendinitis
- Stiff neck, whiplash
- Tennis or golf elbow
- Frozen shoulder
- Trigeminal neuralgia
- Stroke
- Sprains, injuries

Mental or emotional:

- Anxiety
- Depression
- Stress
- Insomnia

Others:

- Increased vitality, stress reduction
- Deep relaxation
- Skin rejuvenation
- Weight control
- Stop smoking
- Alcohol, drugs, and other addictions
- Stronger immune system
- Improved sleeping

How to Find a Practitioner

TCM is the foundation of the many different styles of the medical practice termed *Oriental medicine*. These different styles of practice developed as various countries and cultures, such as Korea, Japan, and even Germany embraced the fundamentals of TCM. A practitioner of TCM is commonly referred to in the United States as an acupuncturist, licensed acupuncturist, acupuncture physician, doctor of acupuncture, doctor of Oriental medicine, or Oriental medical doctor. The titles vary according to the state's licensing regulations. If seeking out a practitioner, look for one that hold's a professional license. If allied health professionals have incorporated any part of Oriental medicine into their practice, such as acupuncture or Chinese herbology, it is recommended that they be certified by or have equivalent education in TCM as outlined by the National Commission for the Certification of Acupuncture and Oriental Medicine (NCCAOM). The minimum competency level should include a specialized education of at least 1,750 hours of study. Many schools throughout the United States have similar curriculums to that of the Chinese schools, and it takes years to attain minimum competency. It is important to remember that TCM is not a development of Western medical science. Many allied health care professionals have legislatively included the practice of acupuncture or Oriental medicine into their scope of practice with little or no training required and have their certifications issued by their own colleagues and professional boards. This is the same as the Board of Acupuncture and Oriental Medicine certifying a practitioner to do surgery, which is clearly absurd. That is why it is important for the consumer to check credentials, certifying agency, and most importantly, length of training before undergoing care.

For information regarding a qualified practitioner in your area, you can contact the National Commission for the Certification of Acupuncture and Oriental Medicine (NCCAOM) at (202) 232-1404; the American Association of Oriental Medicine (AAOM) at (610) 266-1433; in Florida, the Florida State Oriental Medical Association (FSOMA) at (800) 578-4865, or visit its website at www.fsoma.com.

36

Chiropractic

Scott L. Drizin, D.C., M.P.S., F.A.A.B.T., and Ellen C. Drizin, M.S.

THANKS TO establishment of rigorous educational standards, research showing the effectiveness of chiropractic techniques, and a grass roots movement toward more conservative alternative therapies, chiropractic now enjoys more popularity and credibility than ever since its establishment by D. D. Palmer in 1895.

Chiropractors are the most widely sought practitioners for alternative back treatment in the United States,[1] and the primary health care provider for 40 percent of back pain episodes.[2]

Relations between the medical establishment and chiropractic have improved considerably in the past 10 to 20 years. Ninety-nine percent of chiropractors report that they refer patients to medical doctors as needed, and half of medical physicians report that they have made referrals to chiropractors.[3]

In their book *Back Pain: What Works!*, Joseph Kandel, M.D. and David Sudderth, M.D., write "Chiropractic has clearly been validated as a treatment for many musculoskeletal conditions in respected medical journals such as the *British Medical Journal*, in reports from the private sector by such institutions as the Rand Corporation, and more recently by governmental agencies including the U. S. Department of Health and Human Services."[4]

The gain in acceptance and scientific support for spinal manipulation have continued to attract more doctors to the profession. In 1979 there were approximately 20,000 practicing chiropractors in the United States.[5] Fifteen years later, in 1994, there were 50,000.[6] Average chiropractic college enrollment increased 44 percent between 1990 and 1995.[7]

All of these factors—the consistent satisfaction of chiropractic patients, research showing effectiveness of spinal manipulation, the interest of the American public in alternative therapies, and the increase in chiropractic students—should serve to make the 21st century the strongest era yet for chiropractic.

Chiropractic Facts

Unless you've been to a chiropractor, chances are you know very little about what they do. Here are a few tidbits about chiropractic care that might surprise you.

- Chiropractors are trained as "first contact physicians."
- On average, chiropractic training requires more hours of basic and clinical science education than medical training.
- More than 80 percent of American workers in preferred provider organization (PPO), point of service (POS), or conventional insurance plans have some level of chiropractic coverage.
- 92 percent of low back pain chiropractic patients return for chiropractic care if a second episode occurs.

What Is a First Contact Physician?

A first contact physician is trained to recognize and evaluate various health care conditions. Once the physician assesses the patient's symptoms, she or he makes the determination to (1) treat the patient, if it is within the scope of her or his expertise, or (2) refer the patient to another type of physician who specializes in treating the patient's complaints.

Along with medical and osteopathic physicians, chiropractic physicians may be considered first contact doctors. All three types of physicians receive extensive training in how to recognize health care problems throughout the body, and refer patients to the health care provider who can meet their needs. As such, chiropractors are "point of entry" physicians into the health care system.[8]

Scope of Chiropractic

When you visit a chiropractor, her or his first job is to determine whether your problem is within the scope of chiropractic care. According to the American Chiropractic Association (ACA), "Chiropractors provide *conservative management* of *neuromusculoskeletal* disorders and related functional clinical conditions, including, but not limited to, back pain, neck pain, and headaches."[9] Let's take apart that statement.

Neuromusculoskeletal Disorders

Your musculoskeletal system is composed of bones, joints, muscles, tendons, and ligaments. Throughout your body runs a network of nerves that carry electrical signals to every part of your body. Together, this system of nerves, bones, and muscle makes up your neuromusculoskeletal system. Chiropractors specialize in treating disorders of this system.

Disorders of the neuromusculoskeletal system include muscle and tendon strains, ligamentous sprains, nerve root irritation, arthritis, sciatica, and a host of other conditions. When one of these disorders occur, pain, inflammation, and nerve irritation may result. These symptoms may become chronic if not treated promptly. This is where the conservative management aspect of the ACA definition comes in.

Conservative Management

Conservative management means that chiropractors do not use drugs or surgery to treat illnesses or injuries. Instead, they use joint manipulation, physical therapy techniques, nutrition, vitamins, minerals, and herbs to alleviate pain and help resolve injuries.

The most well-known chiropractic treatment is spinal manipulation. The doctor gently palpates your spine and the areas next to it to feel for subluxations (also known as vertebral segmental dysfunction). *Subluxations* are alterations of the normal mechanics between two vertebrae. This alteration may cause the spine to be out of alignment. The misalignment may compromise joint function and range of motion, which can cause muscle spasm, nerve root irritation, pain, and restrict movement.

To correct these subluxations, the chiropractor uses manual manipulation to restore free movement and alleviate pressure on the nerve. Using a quick hand thrust, the chiropractor moves the joint slightly beyond its normal range of motion. Some doctors use devices such as the activator instrument to accomplish a similar goal.

What Else Do Chiropractors Do Besides Manipulate the Spine?

Just as there are philosophical differences within any health care field, differences exist among chirpractors as well. Traditionally, chiropractors have been referred to as either "straights" or "mixers." *Straights* practice spinal manipulation only. *Mixers*, who make up the majority of today's chiropractors, practice spinal manipulation plus provide other types of conservative care as needed. Both mixers and straights agree that the body has an innate ability to heal itself and maintain wellness. The goal, therefore, is to help the patient achieve this wellness through conservative chiropractic care.

In addition to spinal manipulation, mixers treat neuromusculoskeletal disorders throughout the body and perform a variety of other physical and nutritional therapies. Physical therapies include ultrasound, electrical muscle stimulation, hot and cold packs, traction, massage, stretching, and rehabilitative exercises. Nutritional therapies include vitamins, minerals, herbs, and homeopathic remedies to support healing. In fact, chiropractors are required to take nutrition as part of their curriculum, whereas it is an elective course for medical and osteopathic physicians.

Based on state licensing laws, some chiropractors may prescribe or give advice on over-the-counter drugs. Depending on your condition, your chiropractor may recommend one or a combination of these different therapies to restore good health.

What to Expect When You Visit a Chiropractor

Chiropractic physicians use the same standards, techniques, and instruments as other health professionals when conducting physical, neurological, and orthopedic examinations.[10]

When you walk in the door for your first visit to a chiropractic physician, the doctor will ask you to fill out a questionnaire detailing your present complaints and past medical history. The doctor will then interview you and ask specific questions to assess the nature of your problem and whether it falls within the scope of chiropractic care. Afterward, the doctor will give you an exam, which includes the usual diagnostic workup such as vital signs, as well as chiropractically oriented orthopedic and neurological testing. Depending on the results of this initial exam, the doctor may order additional tests such as X rays, MRI, nerve conduction studies, or lab work.

After reviewing all diagnostic results, the doctor will discuss treatment options with you. From a chiropractic perspective, this may include spinal or joint manipulation combined with other forms of physical and nutritional therapies. If necessary, the chiropractor will refer you to other types of specialists, such as neurologists or orthopedists, for consultation or concurrent care.

Musculoskeletal injuries usually require a course of therapy. The exact number of visits is determined by the nature of your disorder and your response to therapy. The goal is to improve your health to the point where treatment is no longer needed or is needed only now and then to maintain your health.

Patient Satisfaction

Patient satisfaction with chiropractic care is high. Low back pain patients consistently report that they are more satisfied with chiropractic care than with medical care.[11] In 92 percent of cases, low back pain patients retain chiropractors as their primary provider when a second incident occurs, compared with 75 percent for general medical practitioners.[12]

Chiropractic Education

At one time the educational standards of chiropractic were not cohesive and therefore widely criticized. In response, the Council on Chiropractic Education (CCE) was established and achieved recognition by the U. S. Department of Education in 1974. The CCE, together with the National Board of Chiropractic Examiners, has established rigorous educational and testing standards for students of chiropractic.

It may surprise you to learn that, on average, chiropractors receive 1,420 hours of basic science education and 3,406 hours of clinical science. This makes 4,826 hours of science education—159 more hours than most medical physicians.[13] But this is only the start. Once the student graduates, the next step is to pass a rigorous set of state licensing board examinations. Forty-seven of fifty states require annual continuing education credits to maintain the license.

Chiropractors may also elect to earn a diplomate in a specialized field. Programs include family practice, applied chiropractic sciences, clinical neurology, orthopedics, radiology, sports injuries, pediatrics, nutrition, rehabilitation, and industrial consulting.

All 16 chiropractic colleges in the United States are now accredited by the CCE. The following chart shows the average number and type of basic and clinical science hours required to graduate with a chiropractic degree.

Average Basic and Clinical Science Hours Required by Chiropractic Colleges[14]

	Hours
Anatomy	570
Biochemistry	150
Microbiology	120
Public Health	70
Physiology	305
Pathology	204
Clinical Science	3,406
Total	4,826

Insurance Coverage

According to a recent review of chiropractic in the United States, "more than 80 percent of American workers in conventional insurance plans, preferred provider organizations, and point-of-service plans now have health insurance that covers at least part of the cost of chiropractic care."[15] HMOs, however, are less likely to provide this type of coverage.

Federal and state programs such as Medicare and Medicaid allow limited coverage. Medicare allows 12 annual visits covering spinal manipulation only. Medicaid and worker's compensation allow basic coverage in most states, but specific benefits vary. Because of insurance equity laws, personal injury protection (PIP) insurance provides coverage on par with all other health care providers in most states.[16]

Choosing a Chiropractor

Choose a chiropractor just as you would any other physician. Look for a physician who is willing to discuss your case in detail, show you the results of imaging and lab testing, and answer your questions thoroughly. The physician should discuss a specific treatment plan with you and keep you abreast of your progress as your care progresses. As with any health care provider, if you are not comfortable with your first choice, shop around for a physician that meets your personal needs.

37

Osteopathic Medicine

Larry Horvath, D.O.

THERE ARE TWO types of medical doctors in the United States: M.D. (allopathic) and D.O. (osteopathic). *Allopathy* is described as disease treated by a morbid reaction, and *osteopathy* is described as any disease of the bone. Both types of physicians are fully licensed to practice medicine and surgery and to prescribe medication in all 50 states.

History

Osteopathic medicine was developed by Andrew T. Still, M.D. (1828–1917). His philosophy centered around the musculoskeletal system and the body's self-healing capacity. He viewed the body as a motor-driven machine. He used mechanical leverage and manipulation of the bones to relieve pressure on the nerves and blood vessels. Proper alignment of nerves, muscle, and bones is required to protect against diseases and also cure diseases. This concept formed the foundation of osteopathic medicine. Today this approach is combined with general scientific medical training and adds an extra dimension to health care.

D.O.s take a holistic approach to the care and treatment of the underlying problem. In keeping with their holistic approach to care, most D.O.s are found in primary care (family and general practice, internal medicine, pediatrics, and obstetrics and gynecology).

Education and Training

Applicants to both D.O. and M.D. colleges have a four-year undergraduate degree. Both complete four years of medical school training. They may then choose to practice in a specialty field of medicine and surgery (such as pediatrics or neurosurgery), typically adding three to six more years of training. The D.O. must be licensed by the state board. Sixty-four percent of all D.O.s remain in primary care practices. Presently 19 osteopathic medical schools exist in the United States.

Today osteopathic physicians continue to be leaders in modern medicine. They combine today's medical technology with the tools of their ears, to listen to their patients; their eyes, to see their patients as whole persons; and their hands, to diagnose and treat injury and illness.

Osteopathic Manipulative Treatment

Osteopathic physicians provide you with the best medicine has to offer. Their knowledge and use of the latest medical technology is complemented by their application of a hands-on treatment tool known as osteopathic manipulation treatment (OMT). This form of manipulation or manual medicine is used to treat a number of disorders of the spine. Using a variety of OMT techniques, the D.O. physician applies manual forces to your body's affected areas to treat the structural abnormalites. This allows specific corrective forces to relieve joint restrictions and misalignments.

Using this modality, people of all ages and backgrounds have found relief from pain. Those who enjoyed the benefits of OMT realize that it can successfully relieve pain and restore mobility. By maintaining proper alignment and structural function, OMT can actually help you avoid injury. Studies have shown that OMT is an effective treatment for acute low back pain.

Sports medicine is also a natural outgrowth of osteopathic practice because of its focus on the musculoskeletal system, manipulative treatment, diet, exercise, and fitness. Many professional sport team physicians are D.O.s.

The D.O. provides you with the best that medicine has to offer. He or she complements the traditional areas of medicine and surgery with the application of OMT.

To contact an osteopathic physician in your area, call the American Osteopathic Association (AOA): American Osteopathic Association, 142 E. Ontario Street, Chicago, IL 60611. (312) 280-5800.

38

Allopathic Medicine: Traditional Western Medicine

Thomas Sultenfuss, M.D.

The medical doctor's role is to prevent, diagnose, and treat diseases and disorders. The treatment protocols may include drugs and surgery as well as dietary and lifestyle regimens. Approximately one-third of all M.D.s are primary care physicians. This includes pediatrics, general internal medicine, and general or family medicine. The other two-thirds of physicians are specialists that are experts in specific fields.

A Brief History

At the beginning of the 19th century medical beliefs were still based on the unchallenged opinions of ancient Greek philosophers and physicians rather than scientific observation and experiment. Many people believed that diseases resulted from an imbalance of essential fluids, or humors: black and yellow bile, blood, and phlegm. This is where we get the terms for such personality types as melancholy, bilious, sanguine, and phlegmatic. Some infections such as malaria and yellow fever were due to miasmas, or "bad air." Blood letting and purging were popular treatments. Almost anyone could claim to be a doctor and set up shop since regulation was virtually nonexistent. From the middle of the 19th century, the character of medicine changed quickly and dramatically as the result of the development of the cell and germ theories. For the first time, large numbers of people were able to prevent and cure once deadly infectious diseases. Emphasis was placed on good public health measures such as sanitation, food, and water systems. Because of the medical and public health measures in the 20th century, life expectancy increased from 45 to 75 years. Medicine is now highly regulated and medical education is intensive.[1]

In less than 175 hundred years, medicine has radically changed. Following is a brief time line showing a few of these changes.[2]

1847 American Medical Association (AMA) was founded. Today the AMA sets the standards for medical ethics, practice, and education. It is an influential voice and advocate for physicians and their patients. It is also the world leader in obtaining, synthesizing, integrating, and disseminating information on health and medical practice.

1849 Ignaz Philipp Semmelweis announced the contagious nature of childbed fever, which killed so many new mothers after delivery.

1860 The Civil War caused a great change in medicine. It was the bloodiest conflict in American history. Almost any injury could be fatal during this period. The bullets were made of unjacketed lead, leaving horrible wounds. Many of these soldiers were left to die where they fell since hospitals seemed only to prolong their agonies. However, this war vastly increased medical and surgical knowledge of trauma and diseases.

1861 Louis Pasteur showed that germs cause decay.

1864 International Red Cross was founded.

1865 Joseph Lister introduced antiseptic surgical technique.

1880s The nursing profession was recognized. Nurses' work included an important role in the patient's treatment as well as in preventive medicine.

1882 Robert Koch discovered the tubercle bacillus.

1897 Ronald Ross discovered the cause of malaria.

1899 Bayer introduced aspirin.

1900 Walter Reed and associates proved the *Aedes aegypti* mosquito transmits yellow fever.

1901 Blood transfusions became available.

In the early 1900s many physicians still didn't understand that infection could be introduced during surgery. Hospitals still remained unsophisticated, poorly funded, and poorly organized. But academics gradually convinced doctors of the link between microbes and disease. Public health authorities learned the importance of modern technology in identifying and controlling infectious agents. States began to monitor food and water for disease-causing microbes. Many new therapies, drugs, and medical technologies had been developed. The government became involved in the medical profession; it set and enforced standards of medical practice and education, leading to licensing of physicians and the reform of medical schools.

1918–1919 The great influenza pandemic killed 15 million people worldwide.

1924 Children were inoculated against tuberculosis (TB).

1930–1945 Antimalarials, sulpha drugs, penicillin, and streptomycin (for tuberculosis) were developed to treat bacterial infections.

1955 Polio vaccine was discovered by Salk.

1963 Vaccine for measles was developed.

1967 Hospice movement was organized for the care of the terminally ill.

1978 First test-tube baby born.

1981 First clinical description of acquired immune deficiency syndrome (AIDS).

As can be seen by the previous time line, the benefits reaped by the world population from the advances of Western medicine are unrivaled. We no longer worry about malaria in Charleston or yellow fever in New Orleans. We let our children swim in public pools without the dread of seeing them die of polio. Whooping cough and diphtheria no longer steal away our babies. These are things we could not take for granted in "the good old days," and they are the direct result of Western medicine's scientific approach to health and disease. Today the field of medicine is still changing rapidly. The quest to prevent and cure disease prevails. Heart disease, cancer, diabetes, and degenerative diseases such as arthritis remain great challenges. Recently physician education has begun to take a serious and long-overdue look at nutrition and alternative medicine disciplines, some of which have been largely ignored or belittled in the past. Hopefully the best of the science and art possessed by each can be synthesized into a more effective approach to medicine.[3]

Education and Training

It takes many years to become an M.D. Requirements include four years of college, four years of medical school, and three to eight years of an internship and residency. A few programs combine the undergraduate years with medical school, reducing the number of years of undergraduate school and medical school by two. There are 125 allopathic medical schools in the United States.

Licensing and Board Certification

An M.D. licensed by the state must graduate from an accredited medical school, pass a licensing exam, and complete one to seven years of postgraduate medical education. In order to be board certified by the American Board of Medical Specialists, a doctor must sit for an exam administered after residency or after having been in practice for a few years. There are 24 different speciality boards.[4]

Part V

Putting It All Together

39

Recommendations

Vitamin and Mineral Dosage Range Table

The following key refers to the vitamin and mineral dosage table on the following pages:

Column 1 identifies the vitamin or mineral and its most bioavailable form(s).

Column 2 states the 1989 recommended daily allowances (RDA) established by the National Research Council.

Column 3 gives the known toxicity levels.

Column 4 is a summary of the scientific data on accepted ranges of vitamins and minerals for a daily multivitamin.

Vitamin and Mineral Dosage Ranges

Vitamin or Mineral	RDA (1989) Women 25+	Toxicity (RDA—1989)	Range
A (Retinol)	4,000 IU	15,000 IU	4,000–15,000 IU
Beta-carotene	——	Unknown	1–15 mg

The 11 most common B vitamins should be taken in a balanced supplement.[A]

Vitamin or Mineral	RDA (1989) Women 25+	Toxicity (RDA—1989)	Range
Thiamine (B1)			
(25 to 50 years)	1.1 mg	Unknown	1.5–200 mg
(51+ years)	1.0 mg		
Riboflavin (B2)			
(25 to 50 years)	1.3 mg	Unknown	1.7–200 mg
(51+ years)	1.2 mg		

Vitamin or Mineral	RDA (1989) Women 25+	Toxicity (RDA—1989)	Range
Niacin (B3) (or niacinamide)			
(25 to 50 years)	15 mg	3–9 g	20–400 mg
(51+ years)	13 mg		
B5 (pantothenic acid)	4–7 mg[B]	10 g	10–300 mg
B6 (pyridoxine)	1.6 mg	117 mg	2–300 mg
B12 (hydroxocobalamin or cyanocobalamin)	2 mcg	Unknown	6–300 mcg
Biotin	30–100 mcg[B]	(none at 10 mg)	25–300 mcg
Choline	—	—	0–100 mg
Folate (folic acid)	180 mcg	(none at 10 mg)	200 mcg–1 mg
Inositol	—	—	80–300 mg
PABA (Para-amino-benzoic acid)	—	—	25–200 mg
C (calcium ascorbate, sodium ascorbate, ascorbic acid)	60 mg	Unknown	60–4,000 mg
D (cholecal-ciferol, or D3)	200 IU	1,000 IU	200–800 IU

Vitamin or Mineral	RDA (1989) Women 25+	Toxicity (RDA—1989)	Range
E (d-alpha-tocopherol acetate, or succinate)	8 mg	More than 3,200 mg	30–800 mg
K (K_1 or K_2)	65 mcg[B]	—	0–100 mcg
CoQ_{10}	—	—	0–200 mg
Boron	—	—	1.5–3 mg
Calcium[C] (calcium citrate, lactate, gluconate)	800 mg	(none at 2,500 mg)	200–1,500 mg
Chromium (picolinate or chromic acetate)	50–200 mcg[B]	—	25–200 mcg
Copper (copper gluconate)	1.5–3 mg[B]	(none at 5–10 mg)	1–3 mg
Iodine (potassium iodide or kelp)	150 mcg	None at 2 mg	25–250 mcg
Iron[D]			
(25–50 years)	15 mg	Unlikely at 75 mg	0–60 mg
(51+ years)	10 mg		
Magnesium[E] (magnesium gluconate, oxide, or sulfate)	280 mg	Unknown	200–1,000 mg

Vitamin or Mineral	RDA (1989) Women 25+	Toxicity (RDA—1989)	Range
Manganese (manganese gluconate)	2.0–5.0 mg[B]	(none at 8–9 mg)	2.5–15 mg
Molybdenum (sodium molybdate)	75–250 mcg[B]	10–15 mg	10–100 mcg
Phosphorous[F]	800 mg (in diet)	—	—
Potassium[G]	—	18 g	—
Selenium	55 mcg[B]	1–5 mg	50–200 mcg
Zinc[H] (zinc gluconate or picolinate)	12 mg	120 mg	12–30 mg

Note: Postmenopausal women require higher doses of pantothenic acid, niacin, calcium, magnesium, manganese, and vitamin K. Iron doses should be reduced.

[A]The B vitamins must be balanced. High doses of individual vitamins have resulted in symptoms of deficiencies in other B vitamins.

[B]For the ninth edition of the RDAS, the NRC subcommittee created the category "Safe and Adequate Intakes" for those nutrients for which there are insufficient data to develop an RDA, but for which there are known potentially toxic upper levels.[1]

[C]General recommendations for premenopausal women and postmenopausal women on ERT/HRT are 800 to 1,000 mg per day. The calcium recommendations for postmenopausal women not taking ERT/HRT are 1,000 to 1,500 mg per day.

[D]Increased ferritin levels and iron levels may cause increased risk of heart disease in postmenopausal women. Certain people are at risk of hemochromatosis, a condition that increases iron absorption and results in failure of many organs. (See Chapter 15.)

[E]The generally accepted supplemental ratio of calcium to magnesium is close to 3 to 1. However, contrary to that is research that suggests a calcium to magnesium ratio of close to 1 to 2.

[F]The generally accepted calcium to phosphorous ratio is 1 to 1. Lower than a 1 to 2 ratio of calcium to phosphorous can reduce blood calcium levels.

[G]No RDA has been given for potassium, but there is an estimated 1,600 to 2,000 mg in the average diet. It is probably best to eat an extra serving of fruits or vegetables daily instead of taking a supplement.

[H]Zinc intakes of 18.5 mg per day have caused impairment of copper status.

Woman's Guide Suggestions for a Vitamin and Mineral Supplement

The *Woman's Guide* Suggestions for a vitamin and mineral supplement, based on current research, should be used only as an informational guide for nonpregnant, healthy women, not a medical recommendation. Consult a physician or registered dietitian to determine the proper nutritional supplement for you.

Women under 40

Vitamin A	5,000 IU	Vitamin Q (CoQ10)	30–50 mg
Beta-carotene	3–5 mg	Boron	3 mg
Thiamin	15 mg	Calcium	1,000–1,500 mcg
Riboflavin	15 mg	Chromium	80 mcg
Niacin	30 mg	Copper	2 mg
B5	25 mg		
B6	50 mg	Iodine	150 mg
Folic acid	400 mcg	Iron	15 mg
B12	50 mcg	Magnesium	400–600 mcg
Biotin	50 mcg	Manganese	5 mg
PABA	30 mg	Molybdenum	15 mcg
Inositol	80 mg	Phosphorus	in diet

Choline	50 mg	Potassium	in diet
Vitamin C	500–1,500 mg	Selenium	50 mcg
Vitamin D	400 IU	Zinc	20 mg
Vitamin E	400–800 mg	Bioflavonoid	100 mg
Vitamin K	10 mcg		

Women over 40

Women over 40 and postmenopausal women require larger amounts of the following nutrients, as listed below.

Niacin	100 mg
Calcium	1,500–2,000 mg
Chromium	100 mcg
Magnesium	500–700 mg
Zinc	30 mg

Iron doses should be reduced to 9 mg.

Woman's Guide Nutritional Guidelines

Nutrients

Sodium: 500 mg to no more than 2,400 per day.

Fat: About 20 percent (certainly less than 30 percent) of total calories with less than 10 percent from saturated fat, reducing hydrogenated fat intake.

Cholesterol: Less than 250 to 300 mg per day.

Complex carbohydrates: 50 to 60 percent of calories.

Fiber: 25 to 30 g per day.

Protein: Less than 15 percent of total calories or 30 to 70 g, relying on fish, legumes, and poultry as protein sources rather than red meat.

Caloric Intake

Women between ages 23 and 50 need approximately 2,200 calories per day and should not drop below 1,200 calories. Women over 50 require approximately 1,900 calories per day. These guidelines are approximations, which will vary depending on physical size (petite versus large-boned) and activity level (couch potato versus triathlete).

Weight

Maintain desirable weight.
Do not yo-yo diet; lose weight slowly if necessary.
Too thin is 15 percent under average weight for age and height.
Too heavy is 30 percent over average weight for age and height.

Exercise

At least three times a week, do both aerobic and weight-bearing exercise.

Foods to Eat

Wide variety of fresh unprocessed foods
Soy products
Fish 1 to 2 times per week or an EPA supplement of 200 to 500 mg per day
Whole grains
Fresh fruits and vegetables
6 to 8 glasses of water per day
Lots of onions and garlic, or take a garlic supplement as directed
Monounsaturated and polyunsaturated oils

Foods to Limit

Alcohol to no more than 1 or 2 drinks per day (if at all)
Sugar to less than 5 tsp per day
Caffeine and chocolate
Saturated oils and fats
Red meats

Things to Try to Avoid

Smoked, salt-cured, and nitrate-cured foods

Processed foods
Hydrogenated oils and fats
Carbonated beverages

Things to Definitely Avoid

Cigarettes
Unnecessary X rays
Direct sun exposure without protective clothing and sunscreen

Vitamins and Minerals

Select a balanced supplement, and take it daily.

Notes

1 Introduction

1. Halbert, Steven C. 1997. Diet and nutrition in primary care. *Complementary and Alternative Therapies in Primary Care*, 24(4):825–840.

2. Knekt, P. et al. 1994. Antioxidant vitamin intake and coronary mortality intake longitudinal population study. *American Journal Epidemiology*, 139:1180–90.

3. Bendich, A., R. Mallick, and S. Leader. 1997. Potential health and economic benefits of vitamin supplementation. *Western Journal of Medicine*, 166:306–12.

2 Vitamins and How to Buy Them

1. Wyngaarden, J. B., L. H. Smith, and J. C. Bennett. 1992. *Cecil textbook of medicine*. Philadelphia: W. B. Saunders Company, 1147.

2. Letter, Penn State Nutritional Center. University Park, PA.

3. Pennington, J. A. T. 1986. Mineral content of foods and total diets: The selected minerals in foods survey, 1982 to 1984. *Journal of the American Dietetic Association*, 86:876–91.

4. Sempos, C. T. et al. 1984. A two-year dietary survey of middle-aged women: repeated dietary records as a measure of usual intake. *Journal of the American Dietetic Association*, 84:1008–13.

5. Hendler, S. S. 1990. *The doctor's vitamin and mineral encyclopedia*. New York: Simon and Schuster, 431.

6. Ibid.

7. Balch, J. E., and P. A. Balch, 1990. Prescription for nutritional healing. New York: Avery, 17.

8. Dunne, L. J. 1990. *Nutrition almanac*. New York: McGraw-Hill, 119–120.

9. Hendler, 430–31.

3 Vitamin A

1. Succari, M. et al. 1991. Influence of sex and age on vitamin A and E status. *Age and Aging* 20:413–416.

2. Harman, D. 1988. Free radicals in aging. *Molecular and Cellular Biochemistry*, 84:155–61.

3. Underwood, B. A. 1991.Vitamin A status and infections. *Nutrition and the M.D.*, 17(9):1–3.

4. Silverman, A. K., C. N. Ellis, and J. J. Voorhees. 1987. Hypervitaminosis A syndrome: A paradigm of retinoid side effects. *Journal of the American Academy of Dermatology*, 16(5):1027–39.

5. Menkes, M. S. et al. 1986. Serum beta-carotene, vitamins A and E, selenium, and the risk of lung cancer. *New England Journal of Medicine*, 315(20):1250–54.

6. Willett, W. C. 1990. Vitamin A and lung cancer. *Nutritional Reviews*, 48(5):201–11.

7. Wyngaarden, J. B., L. H. Smith, and J. C. Bennett, 1992. *Cecil Textbook of Medicine*. Philadelphia: W. B. Saunders, 1178–82.

8. Tavani, A. et al. 1997. Beta-carotene intake and risk of non-fatal acute myocardial infarction in women. *European Journal of Epidemiology*, 13:631–37.

9. Grahm, S. et al. 1991. Nutritional epidemiology of postmenopausal breast cancer in Western New York. *American Journal of Epidemiology*, 134(6):552–66.

10. Zaridze, D. et al. 1991. Diet, alcohol consumption and reproductive factors in a case-control study of breast cancer in Moscow. *International Journal of Cancer*, 48:493–501.

11. Lee, H. P. et al. 1992. Risk factors breast cancer by age and menopausal status: A case-control study in Singapore. *Cancer Causes and Control*, 3:313–22.

12. Lotan, R. 1996. Retinoids in cancer chemoprevention. Federation of American Societies for Experimental Biology, 1031–39.

13. Mayne, S. T., S. Graham, and T. Zheng. 1991. Dietary retinol: Prevention or promotion of carcinogenesis in humans? *Cancer Causes and Control*, 2:443–50.

14. Hislop, T. G. et al. 1986. Childhood and recent eating patterns and risk of breast cancer. *Cancer Detection and Prevention*, 9:47–58.
15. Santamaria, L., M. Dell'Orti, and A. B Santamaria. 1989. Beta-carotene supplementation associated with intermittent retinol administration in the treatment of premenopausal mastodynia. *Boll Chim Farmaceutico*, 128:284–87.
16. Mayne, S. T.
17. Harris, R. W. C. et al. 1991. A case-control study of dietary carotene in men with lung cancer and in men with other epithelial cancers. *Nutrition and Cancer*, 5:63–68.
18. Fontham, E. T. H. 1990. Protective dietary factors and lung cancer. *International Journal of Epidemiology*, 19(3):32–42.
19. Kalandidi, A. et al. 1990. Passive smoking and diet in the etiology of lung cancer among non-smokers. *Cancer Causes and Control*, 1:15–21.
20. Willett, W. C.
21. Heinonen, O. P. et al. 1994. The effect of beta-carotene on the incidence of lung cancer and other cancers in male smokers. *New England Journal of Medicine*, 330:1029–35.
22. Li, J. Y. et al. 1993. Preliminary report on the results of nutrition prevention trials of cancer and other common diseases among residents in Linxian, China. *EBH*, 15(3)165–81.
23. Colditz, G. A. et al. 1985. Increased green and yellow vegetable intake and lowered cancer deaths in an elderly population. *American Journal of Clinical Nutrition*, 41:32–36.
24. Nowak, R. 1994. Beta-carotene: Helpful or harmful? *Science*, 264:500–01.
25. Levine, Norman. et al. Nov. 1997. Trial of retinol and isotretinoin in skin cancer prevention: A randomized, double blind, controlled trial. *Cancer Epidemiology, Bio Markers & Prevention*, 6; 957–61.
26. Moon T. E. et al. 1997. Retinoids in prevention of skin cancer. *Cancer Letters*, 114:203–05.
27. Bosco, D. 1989. The people's guide to vitamins and minerals from A to zinc. Chicago: Contemporary Books, 36.
28. Micozzi, M. S. et al. 1992. Plasma carotenoid response to chronic intake of selected foods and beta-carotene supplements in men. *American Journal of Clinical Nutrition*, 55:1120–25.
29. Perry, S, and K. O'Hanlan, 1992. *Natural Menopause*. Reading: Addison-Wesley, 137.
30. Berg, G., L. Kohlmeier, and H. Brenner, 1997. Use of oral contraceptives and serum beta-carotene. *European Journal of Clinical Nutrition*, 51:181–87.

31. Silverman, A. K.
32. Wyngaarden, 1178–82.
33. Silverman, A. K.
34. Ibid.
35. Costas, K. et al. 1987. Use of supplements containing high-dose vitamin A—New York State, 1983–1984. *Journal of the American Medical Association*, 257(10):1292–97.

4 The B Vitamins

1. Benton, David, Rebecca Griffiths, and Jurg Haller. 1997. Thiamine supplementation mood and cognitive functioning. *Psychopharmacology*, 129:66–71.
2. Suzuki, M., and Y. Itokawa. 1996. Effects of thiamine supplementation on exercise-induced fatigue. *Metabolic Brain Disease*, 11:1.
3. Wyngaarden, J. B., L. H. Smith, and J. C. Bennett. 1992. *Cecil textbook of medicine*. Philadelphia: W. B. Saunders, 1171.
4. Ibid., 1172.
5. Luria, M. H. 1998. Effect of low-dose niacin on high-density lipoprotein cholesterol and total cholesterol/high-density lipoprotein cholesterol ratio. *Archives of Internal Medicine*, 148:2493–95.
6. Carlson, L. A., A. Hamsten, and A. Asplund. 1989. Pronounced lowering of serum levels of lipoprotein Lp(a) in hyperlipidaemic subjects treated with nicotinic acid. *Journal of Internal Medicine*, 226:271–76.
7. Canner, P. L. et al. 1986. Fifteen-year mortality in coronary drug project patients: Long-term benefit with niacin. *Journal of the American College of Cardiology*, 8:1245–55.
8. McKenney, J. M. et al. 1994. A comparison of the efficacy and toxic effects of sustained- vs. immediate-release niacin in hypercholesterolemic patients. *Journal of the American Medical Association*, 271(9):672–77.
9. Wyngaarten, J. B., 1175.
10. Coppola, A., P. G. Brady, and H. J. Nord. 1994. Niacin-induced hepatotoxicity: Unusual presentations. *Southern Medical Journal*, 87(1):30–32.
11. Agte, V. V., K. M. Paknikar, and A. S. A. Chiplonkar. 1997. Effect of nicotinic acid in zinc and iron metabolisms. *BioMetals*, 10:271–76.
12. National Research Council. 1989. *Recommended dietary allowances*. Washington, D.C.: National Academy Press, 172.
13. Folkers, Karl. 1996. Relevance of the biosynthesis of Coenzyme Q10 and the four bases of DNA as a rationale for the molecular causes of cancer

and a therapy. *Biochemical and Biophysical Research Communications*, 224:358–61.

14. Hansen, C., J. Leklem, and L. Miller. 1997. Changes and vitamin B6 status indicators of women fed a constant protein diet with varying levels of vitamin B6. *American Journal of Clinical Nutrition*, 66:1379–87.

15. Dalton, K., and M. J. T. Dalton. 1987. Characteristics of pyridoxine overdose neuropathy syndrome. *Acta Neurologica Scandinvica*, 76:8–11.

16. Morrison, H. I. et al. 1996. Serum folate and risk of fatal coronary heart disease. *Journal of the American Medical Association*, 275:1893–96.

17. Lashner, B. A. et al. 1989. Effect of folate supplementation on the incidence of dysplasia and cancer in chronic ulcerative colitis. *Gastroenterology*, 97:255–59.

18. Lashner, B. A. et al. 1997. The effect of folic supplementation on the risk for cancer or dysplasia in ulcerative colitis. *Gastroenterology*, 112:29–32.

19. Palca, J. 1992. Agencies split on nutritional advice. *Science*, 257:1857.

20. Rush, D. 1994. Periconceptional folate and neural tube defect. *American Journal of Clinical Nutrition*, 59(suppl):511s–16s.

21. Ibid. 1994.

22. Butterworth, C. E. et al. 1982. Improvement in cervical dysplasia associated with folic acid therapy in users of oral contraceptives. *American Journal of Clinical Nutrition*, 35:73–82.

23. Potischman, N. 1993. Nutritional epidemiology of cervical neoplasia. *Journal of Nutrition*, 123:424–29.

24. Ibid.

25. Potischman, Nancy, and Louise Brinton. 1996. Nutrition and cervical neoplasia. *Cancer Causes and Control*, 1:113–26.

26. Joyal, C. C., R. Lalonde, V. Vikis-Freibergs, and I. M. Botez. 1993. Are age-related behavioral disorders improved by folate administration? *Experimental Aging Research*, 19:367–76.

27. Sauberlich, H. E. et al. 1987. Folate requirement and metabolism in nonpregnant women. *American Journal of Clinical Nutrition*, 46:1016–28.

28. Shils, M. E., and V. R. Young. 1998. *Modern nutrition in health and disease*. Philadelphia: Lea & Febiger, 412.

29. Palca.

30. Shojania, A. M. 1975. The effect of oral contraceptives on folate metabolism. III. Plasma clearance and urinary folate excretion. *Journal of Laboratory and Clinical Medicine*, 85(2):185–90.

31. Milne, D. B., W. K. Canfield, J. R. Mahalko, and H. H. Sandstead. 1984. Effect of oral folic acid supplementations on zinc, copper, and iron

absorption and excretion. *American Journal of Clinical Nutrition*, 39:535–39.

32. Teunisse, S. et al. 1996. Dementia subnormal levels of vitamin B_{12}: Effects of replacement therapy on dementia. *Journal Neurology*, 243:522–29.

33. Victor, Herbert. Vitamin B_{12} and folic acid supplementation from letters to the editor. Mount Sinai and Bronx V.A. Medical Centers, 130 West Kingsbride Road, Bronx, NY 10468-3922.

34. Zeisel, S. H. 1992. Choline: an important nutrient in brain development, liver function, and carcinogenesis. Journal of the American College of Nutrition, 11(5):473–81.

35. National Research Council, 264.

36. Shils, 447.

5 Vitamin C

1. Bhambhani, M. M., C. J. Bates, and A. J. Crisp. 1991. Plasma ascorbic acid concentrations in osteoporotic outpatients. *British Journal of Rheumatology*, 31(2):142–43.

2. Dembure, P. P., A. R. Janko, J. H. Priest, and L. J. Elsas. 1987. Ascorbate regulation of collagen biosynthesis in Ehlers-Danlos syndrome, Type VI. *Metabolism*, 36(7):687–91.

3. Thwaites, M., and S. Dean. 1985. Chronic leg ulcers. *Australian Family Physician*, 14(4):292–98.

4. Williams, R. N., C. A. Paterson, K. E. Eakins, and P. Bhattacherjee. 1984. Ascorbic acid inhibits the activity of polymorphonuclear leukocytes in inflamed ocular tissue. *Experimental Eye Research*, 39:261–65.

5. Hemila, H., P. Roberts, and M. Wikstrom. 1984. Activated polymorphonuclear leukocytes consume vitamin C. *Federation of European Biochemical Societies Letters*, 178(1):25–30.

6. Williams, R. N., and C. A. Paterson. 1986. A protective role for ascorbic acid during inflammatory episodes in the eye. *Experimental Eye Research*, 42:211–18.

7. Frei, B., L. England, and B. N. Ames. 1989. Ascorbate is an outstanding antioxidant in human blood plasma. *Proceedings of the National Academy of Science USA*, 86:6377–81.

8. Ten-State Nutritional Survey, 1968–1970, National Health and Nutrition Examination Survey (NHANES I), 1971–1974, studied people from age 3–74; NHANES II, 1976–1980, children 3–11. Hispanic National Health and Nutritional Examination Survey (HNHANES), 1982–1984, for persons 4–74. NHANES I and II were designed to supply health and nutritional information

for civilian, noninstitutionalized populations of the United States. HNHANES was designed to study the same information from three Hispanic populations in Florida, the Southwest, and in Puerto Rico and New York.

9. Enstrom, J. E., L. E. Kanim, and M. A. Klien. 1992. Vitamin C intake and mortality among a sample of the United States population. *Epidemiology*, 3(3):194–202.

10. Ibid.

11. Jacques, P. F. et al. 1997. Long-term vitamin C supplement use and prevalence of early age-related lens opacities. *American Journal of Clinical Nutrition*, 66:911–16.

12. Gey, K. F., H. B. Stahelin, P. Puska, and A. Evans. 1987. Relationship of plasma level of vitamin C to mortality from ischemic heart disease. *Annals of the New York Academy of Science*, 488:110–23.

13. Ness, A. R., J. W. Powles, and K. Khaw. 1996. Vitamins C and cardiovascular disease: A systematic review. *Journal of Cardiovascular Risk*, 3:513–21.

14. Ness, A. R.,, D. Chee, and P. Elliott. 1997. Vitamin C and blood pressure—An overview. *Institute of Public Health*, Cambridge UK, 15(1):343–50.

15. Ness, A. R. et al. 1996. Vitamin C status and the blood pressure. *Journal of Hypertension*, 14(4):503–08.

16. Sahyoun, N. R., P. F. Jaques, and R. M. Russell. 1996. Carotenoids, vitamins C and E, and mortality in an elderly population. *American Journal of Epidemiology*, 144(5):501–11.

17. Erden, F. et al. 1985. Ascorbic acid effect on some lipid fractions in human beings. *Acta Vitaminol Enzymo*l, 7(1–2)131–38.

18. Koumans, A. K. J., and A. J. Wildschut. 1985. Nutrition and atherosclerosis: Some neglected aspects. *Clinical Cardiology*, 8:547–51.

19. Chen, L. H., G. A. Boissonneault, and H. P. Glauert. 1988. Vitamin C, Vitamin E, and Cancer (Review). *Anticancer Research*, 8:739–48.

20. Kyrtopoulos, S. 1987. Ascorbic acid and the formation of N-nitroso compounds: possible role of ascorbic acid in cancer prevention. *American Journal of Clinical Nutrition*, 45:1344–50.

21. Anderson, R., A. J. Theron, and G. J. Ras. 1988. Ascorbic acid neutralizes reactive oxidants released by hyperactive phagocytes from cigarette smokers. *Lung*, 166:149–59.

22. Schwartz, J., and S. T. Weiss. 1994. Relationship between dietary vitamin C intake and pulmonary function in the First National Health and Nutrition Examination Survey (NHANES I). *American Journal of Clinical Nutrition*, 59:1110–14.

23. Romney, S. L. et al. 1985. Plasma vitamin C and uterine cervical dysplasia. *American Journal of Obstetric and Gynecology*, 151:976–80.
24. Pauling, L. 1971. The significance of the evidence about ascorbic acid and the common cold. *Proceedings of the National Academy of Science USA*, 68(11):2678–81.
25. Hemila, H. 1992. Vitamin C and the common cold. *British Journal of Nutrition*, 67:3–16.
26. Karlowski, T. R. et al. 1975. Ascorbic acid for the common cold. *Journal of the American Medical Association*, 231:1038–42.
27. Hemila, Harri. Vitamin C supplementation and common cold symptoms: Problems with inaccurate reviews. *Nutrition*, 12(11/12):804–09.
28. McLindon, T. E. et al. 1996. Do antioxidant the macro nutrients protect against the development and progression of knee osteoarthritis. *Arthritis & Rheumatism*, 39(4):648–56.
29. Soffa, Virginia M. 1996. Alternatives to Hormone Replacement for Menopause. *Alternative Therapies*, 2(2):34-39.
30. Bagchi, B. D. et al. 1997. Oxygen free radical scavenging abilities of vitamins C and E, and a grape seed proanthocyanidin extract in vitro. *Research Communications in Molecular Pathology and Pharmacology*, 95(2):179–89.
31. Podmore, Ian D. et al. 1998. Vitamin C exhibits pro-oxidant properties. *Nature*, 392:659.
32. Herbert, K. E. 1998. Personal communication.
33. Fulghum, D. D. 1977. Ascorbic acid revisited. *Archives of Dermatology*, 113:91–92.
34. Bhambhani, et al. 142–43.
35. Shils, M. E., and V. R. Young. 1988. *Modern nutrition in health and disease*. Philadelphia: Lea & Febiger, 417–35.
36. Ibid.

6 Vitamin D

1. Mortensen, L., and P. Charles. 1996. Bioavailability of calcium supplements and the effect of vitamin D: Comparisons between milk, calcium carbonate, and calcium carbonate plus vitamin D. *American Journal of Clinical Nutrition*, 63:354–57.
2. Lukert, B., J. Higgins, and M. Stoskopf. 1992. Menopausal bone loss is partially regulated by dietary intake of vitamin D. *Calcified Tissue International*, 51:173–79.
3. Ibid.
4. Ibid.

5. Lips, P. et al. 1988. The effect of vitamin D supplementation on vitamin D status and parathyroid function in elderly subjects. *Journal of Clinical Endocrinology and Metabolism*, 67:644–50.

6. Krolner, B. 1983. Seasonal variation of lumbar spine bone mineral content in normal women. *Calcified Tissue Institute*, 35:145–47.

7. Krall, E. A. et al. 1989. Effect of vitamin D intake on seasonal variations in parathyroid hormone secretion in postmenopausal women. *New England Journal of Medicine*, 321:1777–83.

8. Draper, H. H. 1991. Nutrition and Osteoporosis. *Canadian Medical Association Journal*, 144(7):889.

9. Sowers, M. R., R. B. Wallace, and J. H. Lemke, 1985. The association of intakes of vitamin D and calcium with blood pressure among women. *American Journal of Clinical Nutrution*, 42:135–42.

10. Wyngaarden, J. B., L. H. Smith, and J. C. Bennett. 1992. *Cecil Textbook of Medicine*. Philadelphia: W. B. Saunders, 1406.

7 Vitamin E

1. Muller, D. P. R. 1986. Vitamin E—its role in neurological function. *Postgraduate Medical Journal*, 62:107–12.

2. Miller, K. L. 1992. Alternatives to estrogen for menopausal symptoms. *Clinical Obstetrics and Gynecology*, 35(4)884–93.

3. Beard, M., and L. Curtis. 1991. *Menopause and the years ahead.* Tucson: Fisher Books, 155.

4. Perry, S., and K. O'Hanlan. 1992. *Natural menopause*. Reading: Addison-Wesley, 33.

5. Jacobowitz, R. 1993. 150 Most-asked questions about menopause. New York: Hearst Books, 145.

6. Beard, 160.

7. Vorherr, H. 1986. Fibrocystic breast disease: pathophysiology, pathomorphology, clinical picture, and management. *American Journal of Obstetrics and Gynecology*, 154(1):161–79.

8. Ernster, V. L. et al. 1985. Vitamin E and benign breast "disease": A double-blind, randomized clinical trial. *Surgery*, 97(4):490–94.

9. London, R. S. et al. 1985. The effect of vitamin E on mammary dysplasia: A double-blind study. *Obstetrics and Gynecology*, 65(1):104–06.

10. Meyer, E. C. et al. 1990. Vitamin E and benign breast disease. *Surgery*, 107(5):549–51.

11. London, R. S., L. Murphy, and K. E. Kitlowski. 1985. Hypothesis: Breast cancer prevention by supplemental vitamin E. *Journal of the American College of Nutrition*, 4:559–64.

12. Gerber, M. et al. 1989. Relationship between vitamin E and polyunsaturated fatty acids in breast cancer. *Cancer*, 64:2347–53.
13. Kimmick, G. G., A. Bell, and M. Bostick. 1997. Vitamin E and breast cancer: A review. *Nutrition in Cancer*, 27(2):109–17.
14. London, R. S. et al. 1987. Efficacy of alpha-tocopherol in the treatment of the premenstrual syndrome. *Journal of Reproductive Medicine*, 32(6):400–04.
15. Bourne, G. H. 1988. *Sociological and medical aspects of nutrition.* Switzerland: Karger, 170.
16. Li, J.Y. et al. 1993. Preliminary report on the results of nutrition prevention trials of cancer and other common diseases among residents in Linxian, China. *EBH*, 15(3)165–81.
17. Menkes, M. S. et al. 1986. Serum beta-carotene, vitamin A and E, selenium, and the risk of lung cancer. *New England Journal of Medicine*, 315:1250–54.
18. Evans, W. J. 1992. Exercise, nutrition and aging. *Journal of Nutrition*, 122:796–801.
19. Van Der Beek, E. J. 1991. Vitamin supplementation and physical exercise performance. *Journal of Sports Science*, 9:77–89.
20. Dekkers, C. et al. 1996. The Roles of antioxidant vitamins and enzymes in the prevention of exercise-induced muscle damage. *Sports Medicine*, 21(3):213–38.
21. Jandak, J., M. Steiner, and P. D. Richardson. 1989. Alpha-tocopherol, an effective inhibitor of platelet adhesion. *Blood*, 73(1):141–49.
22. Stephens, N. G. et al. 1996. The random minus to control trial of vitamin E in patients with coronary disease: Cambridge heart antioxidant study(CHAOS). *Lancet*, 347:781–86.
23. Diplock, A. T. 1997. Will the 'good fairies' please prove to us that vitamin E lessens human degenerative disease? *Free Radical Research*, 26:565–83.
24. Rimm, E. B., and M. J. Stampfer. 1997. The roll of antioxidants in preventive cardiology. *Current Opinion in Cardiology*, 12:188–94.
25. Olsson, A. G., and X. M. Yuan. 1996. The antioxidants in the prevention of atherosclerosis. *Current Opinion in Lipidology*, 7:374–80.
26. Stampfer, M. J. et al. 1993. Vitamin E. consumption and the risk of coronary disease in women. *New England Journal of Medicine*, 328:1444–49.
27. Cockcroft, J., and P. Chowienczyk. 1996. Beyond cholesterol reduction in coronary heart disease: Is vitamin E the answer. *Heart*, 76:293–94.
28. Epstein, F. H. 1997. Antioxidants and atherosclerosis heart disease. *New England Journal of Medicine*, 337(6):408–16.

29. Meyer, F., I. Bairati, and G. R. Dagenais. 1996. Lower ischemic heart disease incidence and mortality among vitamin supplement users. *Canadian Journal of Cardiology*, 12(10):930–34.

30. Poltnick, G. D. et al. 1997. Effect of antioxidant vitamins on the transient impairment of endothelium-dependent brachial artery vasoactivity following a single high-fat meal. *Journal of the American Medical Association*, 278:1682–86.

31. Kwasniewska, A., A.Tukendorf, and M. Semezuk, 1997. Content of alpha-tocopherol in blood serum of the human papillomavirus-infected women with cervical dysplasia. *Nutrition and Cancer*, 28(3): 248–51.

32. Sano, Mary et al. 1997. A Controlled trial of selegiline, alpha-tocopherol, or both as a treatment for alzheimer's disease. *New England Journal of Medicine*, 336:1216–22.

33. Bässler, K. H. 1991. On the problematic nature of vitamin E requirements: Net vitamin E. *Z Ernährungswiss*, 30:174–80.

34. Wyngaarden, J. B., H. L. Smith, and J. C. Bennett. 1992. *Cecile Textbook of Medicine*. Philadelphia: W. B. Saunders, 1181.

35. Hendler, S. S. 1990. *The doctor's vitamin and mineral encyclopedia*. New York: Simon and Schuster, 108.

36. Bendich, A., and L. J. Machlin. 1988. Safety of oral intake of vitamin E1, 2. *American Journal of Clinical Nutrition*, 48:612–19.

37. Ibid.

38. Wyngaarden, 1181.

39. Halbert, Steven C. 1997. Diet and nutrition in primary care. *Complementary and Alternative Therapies in Primary Care*, 24(4): 825–40.

8 Vitamin K

1. Knapen, M. H. J., K. Hamulyák, and C. Vermeer. 1989. The effect of vitamin K supplementation on circulating osteocalcin (bone Gla protein) and urinary calcium excretion. *Annals of Internal Medicine*, 111:1001–05.

2. Tomita, A. 1971. Postmenopausal osteoporosis Ca study with vitamin K_2. *Clinical Endocrinology*, 19:731–36.

3. Hart, J. P. et al. 1984. Circulating vitamin K_1 levels in fractured neck of femur. *Lancet*, 2:283.

4. Hodges, S. J. et al. 1991. Depressed levels of circulating menaquinones in patients with osteoporotic fractures of the spine and femur neck. *Bone*, 12:387–89.

5. Kanai, T. et al. 1997. Serum vitamin K level and bone mineral density and post menopausal women. *International Journal of Gynecology & Obstetrics*, 56:25–30.

6. Hamulyák, K., and C. Vermeer. 1985. Osteocalcin: A vitamin K dependent protein in bone. *Netherlands Journal of Medicine*, 28:305–06.

7. Uchida, K., and T. Komeno, 1988. Relationships between dietary and intestinal vitamin K, clotting factor levels, plasma vitamin K, and urinary Gla in Vitamin K: *Current advances in vitamin K research*. John W. Suttie, ed., New York: Elesvier, 491.

8. Jie, K. S. G. et al. 1996. Vitamin K status and bone mass in women with and without aortic atherosclerosis: A population-based study. *Calcified Tissue International*, 59:352–56.

9. Hodges, 387–89.

10. Hendler, S. S. 1990. The doctors vitamin and mineral encyclopedia. New York: Simon and Schuster, 109–11.

11. Uchida.

12. Shils, M. E., and V. R. Young, 1988. *Modern nutrition in health and disease*. Philadelphia: Lea & Febiger, 735.

13. National Research Council. 1989. *Recommended dietary allowances*. Washington D.C.: National Academy Press, 112.

9 CoQ_{10}

1. Folkers, Karl. 1996. Relevance of the biosynthes of coenzyme Q and of the four bases of DNA as a rationale for the molecular causes of cancer and a therapy. *Biochemical and Biophysical Research Communications*, 224:358–61.

2. Thomas, Shane R., and Roland Stocker. 1996. Cosupplementation with co-enzyme Q prevents the prooxidant effect of alpha tocopherol and increases the resistance of LDL to transition metal-dependent oxidation initiation. *Arteriosclerosis, Thrombosis, and Vascular Biology*, 16(5):687–96.

3. Thomas, Shane R., Jiri Neuzil, and Roland Stocker. 1997. Inhibition of LDL oxidation by Ubiquinol-10. A protective mechanism for coenzyme Q in atherogenesis? *Molecular Aspects of Medicine*, 18:85–103.

4. Bargossi, A. M., M. Battino, et al. 1994. Exogenous CoQ_{10} preserves plasma ubiquinone levels in patients treated with 3-hydroxy-3-methylglutaryl coenzyme A reductase inhibitors. *International Journal of Clinical Laboratory Research*, 24(3):171–76.

5. Folkers, K., P. Langsjoen, et al. 1990. Lovastatin decreases coenzyme Q levels in humans. *Proceedings of the National Academy of Sciences U.S.A.*, 87:8931–34.

6. Folkers, K., S. Vadhanavikit, and S. A. Mortensen. 1985. Biochemical rationale and myocardial tissue data on the effective therapy of cardiomyopathy with coenzyme Q_{10}. *Proceedings of the National Academy of Sciences U.S.A.*, 82(3):901–04.

7. Morisco, C., B. Trimarco, and M. Condorelli. 1986. Effects of coenzyme Q_{10} therapy in patients with congestive heart failure: A long-term, multicenter, randomized study. Seventh international symposium on biomedical and clinical aspects of coenzyme Q. Folkers, K. et al., eds. *The Clinical Investigator*, 71:S134–36.

8. Langsjoen, P. H., S. Vadhanavikit, and K. Folkers. 1985. Response of patients in classes III and IV of cardiomyopathy to therapy in a blind and crossover trial with coenzyme Q_{10}. *Proceedings of the National Academy of Sciences U.S.A.*, 82:4240–44,.

9. Mortensen, S. A. et al. 1990. Coenzyme Q_{10}: Clinical benefits with biochemical correlates suggesting a scientific breakthrough in the management of chronic heart failure. *International Journal of Tissue Reaction*, 12(3):155–62.

10. Langsjoen, P .H. et al. Treatment of essential hypertension with Coenzyme Q_{10}. Eighth annual symposium on biomedical and clinical aspects of coenzyme Q. *The Molecular Aspect of Medicine*, 15(Supplement):S265–72.

11. Kuklinski, B., E. Weissenbacher, and A. Fahnrich. 1994. Coenzyme Q_{10} and antioxidants in acute myocardial infarction. *Molecular Aspects of Medicine*, 15(Supplement):S143–47.

12. Langsjoen, P. H. 1998. Personal communication.

13. Willis, R. 1998. Personal communication.

14. Folkers, Karl.

15. Lockwood, K., S. Moesgard, and K. Folkers. 1994. Partial and complete regression of breast cancer in patients in relation to dosage of coenzyme Q_{10}. *Biochemical and Biophysical Research Communications*, 199(3):1504–08.

16. Ylikosky, T. et al. 1997. The effect of coenzyme Q_{10} on the exercise performance of cross-country skiers. *Molecular Aspects of Medicine*, 18SUPPL:S283–90.

17. Langsjoen, P. H. 1994. Introduction to Coenzyme Q_{10}. Private publication.

18. National Research Council. 1989. *Recommended dietary allowances.* Washington D.C.: National Academy Press, 263.

10 Boron

1. Volpe, S. L., J. Taper, and S. Meacham. 1993. The relationship between boron and magnesium status and bone mineral density in the human: A review, *Magnesium Research*, 6(3):291–96.

2. Shils, M. E., and V. R. Young. 1998. Modern nutrition in health and disease. Philadelphia: Lea & Febiger, 282.

3. Nielsen, F. H. et al. 1987. Effect of dietary boron on mineral, estrogen, and testosterone in metabolism in postmenopausal women. *FASEB Journal*, 1:394–97.

11 Calcium

1. Amschler, D. H. 1985. Calcium Intake: A lifelong proposition. *Journal of School Health*, 55(9):360–63.

2. Ibid.

3. Mayes, K. 1986. Osteoporosis: Brittle bones and the calcium crisis. Santa Barbara: Pennant Books, 80–81.

4. Halbert, Steven C. 1997. Diet and nutrition in primary care. *Complementary and Alternative Therapies in Primary Care*, 24(4):825–40.

5. Tesar, R. et al. 1992. Axial and peripheral bone density and nutrient intakes of postmenopausal vegetarian and omnivorous women. *American Journal of Clinical Nutrition*, 56:699–704.

6. Tylavsky, F. A., and J. B. Anderson. 1988. Dietary factors in bone health of elderly lacto-ovovegetarians and omnivorous women. *American Journal of Clinical Nutrition*, 48:842–49.

7. Hunt, I. F. et al. 1989. Bone Mineral content in postmenopausal women: Comparison of omnivorous and vegetarians. *American Journal of Clinical Nutrition*, 50:517–23.

8. Ellis, F. R., S. Holesh, and J. W. Ellis. 1972. Incidence of osteoporosis in vegetarians and omnivorous. *American Journal of Clinical Nutrition*, 25:555–58.

9. Marsh, A. G. et al. 1980. Cortical bone density of adult lacto-ovo-vegetarian and omnivorous women. *Journal of the American Dietetic Association*, 76:148–51.

10. Soffa, Virginia M. 1996. Alternatives to hormone replacement for menopause. *Alternative Therapies*, 2(2):34–39.

11. Angus, R. M. et al. 1988. Dietary intake and bone density. *Bone and Mineral*, 4:265–77.

12. Bernstein, D. S. et al. 1966. Prevalence of osteoporosis in high- and low-fluoride areas in North Dakota. *Journal of the American Medical Association*, 198(5):85–90.

13. Simonen, O., and O. Laitinen. 1985. Does fluoridation of drinking water prevent bone fragility and osteoporosis? *Lancet*, (August):432–34.
14. Mamelle, N. et al. 1998. Risk-benefit ratio of sodium fluoride treatment in primary vertebral osteoporosis. *Lancet*, (August):361–65.
15. Renner, R. P., L. J. Boucher, and H. W. Kaufman. 1984. Osteoporosis in postmenopausal women. *Journal of Prosthetic Dentistry*, 52(4):581–88.
16. Salisbury, J. J., and J. E. Mitchell. 1991. Bone mineral density and anorexia nervosa in women. *American Journal of Psychiatry*, 148:768–74.
17. Freudenheim, J. L., N. E. Johnson, and E. L. Smith. 1986. Relationships between usual nutrient intake and bone-mineral content of women 35–65 years of age: longitudinal and cross-sectional analysis. *American Journal of Clinical Nutrition*, 44:863–76.
18. Bostick, R. 1997. Human studies of calcium supplementation and colorectal epithelial cell proliferation. *Cancer Epidemiology, Biomarkers & Prevention*, 6:971–80.
19. Martinez, M. L. 1996. Calcium, vitamin D and that occurrence of colo-rectal cancer among women. *Journal of the National Cancer Institute*, (19):1375–82.
20. Yang, C. et al. 1997. Calcium and magnesium in drinking water and risk of death from colon cancer. *Japanese Journal of Cancer Research*, 88:928–33.
21. White, E., J. Shannon, and R. E. Patterson. 1997. Relationship between vitamin and calcium supplement use and cancer. *Cancer Epidemiology, Biomarkers & Prevention*, 6:769–74.
22. Holbrook, T. L., and E. Barrett-Connor. 1991. Calcium intake: Covariates and confounders. *American Journal of Clinical Nutrition*, 53:741–44.
23. Garland, C. et al. 1985. Dietary vitamin D and calcium and risk of colorectal cancer: A 19-year prospective study in men. *Lancet*, (February):307-25.
24. Sowers, M. R., R. B. Wallace, and J. H. Lemke. 1985. The association of intakes of vitamin D and calcium with blood pressure among women. *American Journal of Clinical Nutrition*, 42:135–42.
25. Angus, 265–77.
26. Dawson-Hughes, B. 1991. Calcium supplementation and bone loss: A review of controlled clinical trials. *American Journal of Clinical Nutrition*, 54:274–80.
27. Reid, I. R. et al. 1993. Effect of calcium supplementation on bone loss in postmenopausal women. *New England Journal of Medicine*, 328(7):460–64.
28. Prince, R. 1993. The calcium controversy revisited: Implications of new data. *Medical Journal of Australia*, 159:404–07.

29. Suleimanm, S. et al. 1997. Effect of calcium intake and physical activity level on bone mass and turnover in healthy, white, postmenopausal women. *American Journal of Clinical Nutrition*, 66: 937–43.

30. Whiting, Susan J. 1997. Calcium supplementation. *Pharmacology Update*, 9(4):187–92.

31. National Research Council. 1989. *Recommended dietary allowances*. Washington, D.C.: National Academy Press, 174–84.

32. Dawson-Hughes, S. S., F. H. Seligson, and V. A. Hughes. 1986. Effects of calcium carbonate and hydroxyapatite on zinc and iron retention in postmenopausal women. *American Clinical Journal*, 44(1):83–88.

12 Chromium

1. Mertz, W. 1993. Chromium in human nutrition: A review. *Journal of Nutrition*, 123:626–33.

2. Anderson, R. A. et al. 1987. Effects of supplemental chromium on patients with symptoms of reactive hypoglycemia. *Metabolism*, 36(4):351–55.

3. Clausen, J. 1988. Chromium induced clinical improvement in symptomatic hypoglycemia. *Biological Trace Element Research*, 17:229–36.

4. Anderson, R. A. 1997. Elevated intakes of supplemental chromium improve glucose and insulin variables in individuals with type 2 diabetes. *Diabetes*, 46:1786–91.

5. Anderson, R. A. 1997. Nutritional factors influencing the glucose/insulin system: Chromium. *Journal of the American College of Nutrition*, 16(5):404–10.

6. Mossop, R. T. 1991. Trivalent chromium, in atherosclerosis and diabetes. Central African Journal of Medicine, 37(11)369–74.

7. Simonoff, M. 1984. Chromium deficiency and cardiovascular risk. *Cardiovascular Research*, 18:591–96.

8. Mertz, 626–33.

9. Mossop, 369–74.

10. Anderson, R. A. 1986. Chromium metabolism and its role in disease processes in man. *Clinical Physiology and Biochemistry*, 4:31–41.

11. Mertz, W. Personal communication.

12. Anderson, R. A. 1997. Chromium as an essential nutrient for humans. *Regulatory Toxicology and Pharmacology*, 26:35-41.

13 Copper

1. Hendler, S. S. 1990. *The doctor's encyclopedia of vitamins and minerals*. New York: Simon and Schuster, 128.

2. Margalioth, E. J., J. G. Schenker, and M. Chevion. 1983. Copper and zinc levels in normal and malignant tissue. *Cancer*, 52:868–72.

3. Brandes, J. M., A. Lightman, A. Drugan, O. Zinder, A. Cohen, and J. Itskovtiz. 1983. The diagnostic value of serum copper/zinc ratio in gynecological tumors. *Acta Obstet Gynecol Scand*, 62:225–29.

4. Kies, C., and J. M. Harms. Copper absorption as affected by supplemental calcium, magnesium, manganese, selenium and potassium. *University of Nebraska Journal* Article Series No. 8965, 45–58.

5. National Research Council. 1989. *Recommended dietary allowances*. Washington, D.C.: National Academy Press, 224–30.

14 Iodine

1. Philips, D. I. W., J. H. Lazarus, and R. Hall. 1988. Iodine metabolism and the thyroid. *Journal of Endocrinology*, 119:361–63.

2. Iodine relieves pain of fibrocystic breasts. *Medical World News*. (January 11, 1988):25.

3. Ghent, W. R., B. A. Eskin, D. A. Low, and L. P. Hill, 1993. Iodine replacement in fibrocystic disease of the breast. *Canadian Journal of Surgery*, 36(5):453–60.

4. National Research Council. 1989. *Recommended dietary allowances*. Washington, D.C.: National Academy Press, 216.

15 Iron

1. Budoff, P. W. 1983. *No more hot flashes*. New York: Warner Books, 268.

2. Lauffer, R. B. 1991. *Iron Balance*. New York: St. Martin's Press, 27-28.

3. Lauffer, 150.

4. Myers, D. G. 1996. The iron hypothesis—does iron cause atherosclerosis? *Clinical Cardiology*, 19:925–29.

5. Sempos, C. T. et al. 1996. Iron and heart disease: The epidemiology data. *Nutrition Reviews*, 54(3):73–84.

6. Corti, M. et al. 1997. Iron status and risk of cardiovascular disease. *Annals of Epidemiology*, 7(1):62–68.

7. Naimark, B. J. 1996. Serum ferritin and heart disease: The effect of moderate exercise on stored iron levels in postmenopausal women. *Canadian Journal of Cardiology*, 12(12):1253–57.

8. Hershko, C., T. E. A. Peto, and D. J. Weatherall. 1988. Iron and infection. *British Medical Journal*, 296:660–64.

9. Dallman, P. R. 1987. Iron deficiency and the immune response. *American Journal of Clinical Nutrition*, 46:329–34.

16 Magnesium

1. National Research Council. 1989. *Recommended dietary allowances*. Washington, D.C.: National Academy Press, 188.

2. McLean, R. M. 1994. Magnesium and its therapeutic uses: A review. *American Journal of Medicine*, 96:63–76.

3. White, J. R., and R. K. Campbell. 1993. Magnesium and diabetes: A review. *Annals of Pharmacotherapy*, 27:775–80.

4. Wyngaarden, J. B., L. H. Smith, and J. C. Bennett. 1992. *Cecil textbook of medicine*. Philadelphia: W. B. Saunders, 1138.

5. National Research Council, 189–90.

6. Halbert, Steven C. 1997. Diet and nutrition in primary care. *Complementary and Alternative Therapies in Primary Care*, 24(4):825–40.

7. Ibid.

8. Stanton, M. F., and F. L. Lowenstein. 1987. Serum magnesium in women during pregnancy, while taking contraceptives, and after menopause. *Journal of the American College of Nutrition*, 6(4):313–19.

9. Schlemmer, A., J. Podenphant, B. J. Riis, and C. Christiansen. 1991. Urinary magnesium in early postmenopausal women. *Magnesium Trace Elements*, 92(10):34–39.

10. Abraham, G. E., and H. Grewal. 1990. A total dietary program emphasizing magnesium instead of calcium. *Journal of Reproductive Medicine*, 35:503–07.

11. Sjogren, A., L. Edvinsson, and B. Fallgren. 1989. Magnesium deficiency in coronary artery disease and cardiac arrhythmias. *Journal of Internal Medicine*, 226:213–22.

12. Dubey, A., and R. Solomon. 1989. Magnesium, myocardial ischaemia and arrhythmias: The role of magnesium in myocardial infarction. *Drugs*, 37:1–7.

13. Teo, K. K., and S. Yusuf. 1993. Role of magnesium in reducing mortality in acute myocardial infarction. *Drugs*, 46(3):347–59.

14. Ibid.

15. Hendler, S. S. 1990. The doctor's vitamin and mineral encyclopedia. New York: Simon and Schuster, 158-59.

16. Itoh, K., T. Kawaski, and M. Nakamura. 1997. The effects of high oral magnesium supplementation on blood pressure, serum lipids and related variables in apparently healthy Japanese subjects. *British Journal of Nutrition*, 78:737–50.

17. Paolisso, G., and M. Barbagallo. 1997. Hypertension, diabetes mellitus, and insulin resistance. *American Journal of Hypertension*, 10:346–55.

18. Bosco, Dominick. 1989. The people's guide to vitamins and minerals from A to zinc. Chicago: Contemporary Books, 248.

17 Manganese

1. Raloff, J. 1986. Reasons for boning up on manganese. *Science News*, 130(13):199.

2. Free-Graves, J. et al. 1990. Manganese status of osteoporotics and age-matched, healthy women. *FASEB Journal*, 4, A777.

3. Johnson, P .E. 1994. Manganese and iron metabolism. *Manganese in Health and Disease*. D. J. Klimas-Tvantzis, ed. Boca Raton: CRC Press, 133–43.

18 Molybdenum

1. Sardesai, V. M. 1993. Molybdenum: An essential trace element. *Mayo Clinic Proceedings*, 8(6):277–81.

19 Phosphorus

1. National Research Council. 1989. *Recommended dietary allowances*. Washington, D.C.: National Academy Press, 186.

2. Ibid.

20 Potassium

1. Khaw, K., and E. Barrett-Connor. 1987. Dietary potassium and stroke-associated mortality. *New England Journal of Medicine*, 316:235–40.

2. National Research Council. 1989. *Recommended dietary allowances*. Washington, D.C.: National Academy Press, 256.

21 Selenium

1. Editors of Prevention Magazine. 1984. *Understanding vitamins and minerals*. Emmaus: Rodale Press, 124-25.

2. Kok, F. J. et al. 1989. Decreased selenium levels in acute myocardial infarction. *Journal of the American Medical Association*, 261(8):1161–64.

3. Oster, O. et al. 1986. The serum selenium concentration of patients with acute myocardial infarction. *Annals of Clinical Research*, 18:36–42.

4. Huttunen, J. K. 1997. Selenium and cardiovascular diseases—An update. *Biomedical and Environmental Sciences*, 10:220–26.

5. Kuklinski, B., E. Weissenbacher, and A. Fahnrich. 1994. Coenzyne Q10 and antioxidants in acute myocardial infarction. *Molecular Aspects of Medicine*, 15Suppl:s143–47.

6. Bourne, G. H. 1988. *Sociological aspects of nutrition*. Basel: Karger, 145–46.

7. Salonen, J. T. et al. 1985. Risk of cancer in relation to serum concentrations of selenium and vitamins A and E: matched case-control analysis of prospective data. *British Medical Journal*, 290:417–20.

8. Koskinen, T. et al. 1987. Serum selenium, vitamin A, vitamin E, and cholesterol concentrations in Finnish and Japanese postmenopausal women. *International Journal for Vitamin and Nutrition Research*, 57:111–14.

9. Salonen, J. T. et al.

10. National Research Council. 1989. *Recommended dietary allowances*. Washington, D.C.: National Academy Press, 218.

11. Shils, M. E., and V. R. Young. 1988. *Modern nutrition in health and disease*. Philadelphia: Lea & Febiger, 266.

12. National Research Council, 221.

22 Zinc

1. Hendler, S. S. 1990. *The doctor's encyclopedia of vitamins and minerals*. New York: Simon and Schuster, 195–96.

2. Miline, D. B. et al. 1987. Ethanol metabolism in postmenopausal women fed a diet marginal in zinc. *American Journal of Clinical Nutrition*, 46:688–93.

3. Halbert, Steven C. 1997. Diet and nutrition in primary care. *Complementary and Alternative Therapies in Primary Care*, 24(4):825–40.

4. Ibid.

5. McClain, C. J., and L. Su. 1983. Zinc deficiency in the alcoholic: A review. *Clinical and Experimental Research*, 7(1):5–10.

6. Chilvers, D. C. et al. 1985. Effects of oral ethinyl oestradiol and norethisterone on plasma copper and zinc complexes in post-menopausal women. *Hormone and Metabolic Research*, 17:532–35.

7. Halbert, Steven C.

8. National Research Council. 1989. *Recommended dietary allowances.* Washington, D.C.: National Academy Press, 210–11.

23 Bones

1. Cooper, K. H. 1989. *Preventing osteoporosis.* New York: Bantam Books, 31–32.

2. Sabatier, J. P. et. al.. 1996. Bone mineral acquisition during adolescence and early adulthood: A study in 574 healthy females 10–24 years of age. *Osteoporosis International*, 6(2):141–48.

3. Theintz, G. et. al. 1992. Longitudinal monitoring of bone mass accumulation in healthy adolescents: Evidence for a marked reduction after 16 years of age at the level of lumbar spine and femoral neck in female subjects. *Journal of Endocrinology and Metabolism*, 75(4):1060–65.

4. Ibid.

5. Fraser, William, D. 1997. Bone preservations and the menopause. *British Journal of Hospital Medicine*, 57(5):212–14.

6. Bowman, M. A., and J. G. Spangler. 1997. Osteoporosis in women. *Primary Care, the 21*(1):27–35.

7. Lee, John R., and Virginia Hopkins. 1996. *What Your Doctor May Not Tell You About Menopause.* Warner Books.

8. Brown, S. E. 1988. Osteoporosis: sorting fact from fallacy. *The Network News*, (July/August).

9. Christiansen, C. 1992. Prevention and treatment of osteoporosis: A review of current modalities. *Bone*, 13:35–39.

10. Rubin, C. G. 1991. Southwestern internal medicine conference: Age-related osteoporosis. *American Journal of Medical Science*, 301(4):281–98.

11. Ettinger, B. 1988. A practical guide to preventing osteoporosis. *Western Journal of Medicine*, 149:691–95.

12. Lindsay, R. 1992. Osteoporosis: *A guide to diagnosis, prevention, and treatment.* National Osteoporosis Foundation. New York: Raven Press.

13. Ibid.

14. Bass, K. M., and T. L. Bush. 1991. Estrogen therapy and cardiovascular risk in women. *Journal*, 143:33–39.

15. Rubin.

16. Lindsay.
17. Wolf, S. M. 1991. *Women's health alert.* Reading: Addison-Welsey, 205.
18. Rubin.
19. Roberts, W. E. et al. What are the risk factors of osteoporosis? National Institute of Dental Research. Grant # DEO9237, 59–62.
20. Renner, R. P., L. J. Boucher, and H. W. Kaufman. 1984. Osteoporosis in postmenopausal women. *Journal of Prosthetic Dentistry*, 52(4):581–88.
21. Cutler, W. B. and C. R. Garcia. 1983. *Menopause: A guide for women and the men who love them.* New York: W. W. Norton, 95.
22. Amschler, D. H. 1985. Calcium intake: A lifelong proposition. *Journal of School Health*, 55(9):360–63.
23. Gutin, B., and M. J. Kasper. 1992. Can vigorous exercise play a role in osteoporosis prevention? *Osteoporosis International*, 2:55–69.
24. Smith, E. L. et al. 1989. Deterring bone loss by exercise intervention in premenopausal and postmenopausal women. *Calcified Tissue International*, 44:312–21.
25. Grove, K. A., and B. R. Londeree. June 1992. Bone density in postmenopausal women: High impact vs. low impact exercise. *Medicine and Science in Sports and Exercise*, 1190–94.
26. Krall, E. A., and B. Dawson-Hughes. 1994. Walking is related to bone density and rates of bone loss. *American Medical Journal*, 96:20–26.
27. Sinaki, M. et al. 1989. Efficacy of nonloading exercises in prevention of vertebral bone loss in postmenopausal women: A controlled trial. *Mayo Clinic Proceedings*, 64:762–69.
28. Levin.
29. Salamone, L. M. et al. 1996. Determinants of pre-menopausal bone mineral density: The interplay of genetic and lifestyle factors. *Journal of Bone and Mineral Research*, 11(10):1557–64.
30. Ulrich, C. M. et al. 1996. Bone mineral density in mother-daughter pairs: Relations to lifetime exercise, lifetime milk consumption, and calcium supplements. *American Journal of Clinical Nutrition*, 63:72–79.
31. Rubin.
32. Marcus, R. et al. 1992. Osteoporosis and exercise in women. *Medicine and Science in Sports and Exercise*, 24(6):301–07.
33. Suleimanm, S. et al. 1997. Effect of calcium intake and physical activity level on bone mass and turnover in healthy, white, postmenopausal women. *American Journal of Clinical Nutrition*, 66:937–43.
34. Kanis, J. A., and R. Passmore. 1989. Calcium supplementation of the diet: Not justified by the present evidence. *British Journal of Medicine*, 298:137–40.

35. Nordin, B. E. C., and R. P. Heaney. 1990. Calcium supplementation of the diet: Justified by present evidence. *British Journal of Medicine*, 300:1056–62.

36. Cummings, R. G. et al. 1997. Calcium intake and fracture risk: Results from the study of osteoporotic fractures. *American Journal of Epidemiology*, 145(10):962–34.

37. Seeman, E. 1997. Osteoporosis: Trials and relations. *The American Journal of Medicine*, three (2A):74s–87s.

38. Scopacasa, F. et al. 1998. Calcium supplementation suppresses bone resorption in early postmenopausal women. *Calcified Tissue International*, 62:8–12.

39. Whiting, Susan J. 1997. Calcium supplementation. *Pharmacology Update*, 9(4):187–92.

40. Holick, M. F. 1996. Vitamin D and bone health. *Journal Nutrition*, 126:1159s–64s.

41. Prince, R. L. 1997. Diet and the prevention of osteoporotic fractures. *New England Journal of Medicine*, 337(10):701–02.

42. Dawson-Hughes, Bess et al. 1997. Effect of calcium and vitamin D supplementation on bone density in men and women 65 years of age or older. *New England Journal of Medicine*, 337(10), 670–76.

43. Thekkinen, M. et al. 1998. Affects the postmenopausal hormone replacement therapy with and without Vitamin D3 on circulating levels of 25-hydroxyvitamin D and 1,25-dihydroxyvitamin D. *Calcified Tissue International*, 62:26–30.

44. Gambacciani, M. et al. 1997. Effects of combined low doses of the isoflavones derivative ipriflavone and estrogen replacement on bone mineral density and metabolism in postmenopausal women. *Maturitas*, 28:75–81.

45. Cooper, C. et al. 1996. Dietary protein intake and bone mass in women. *Calcified Tissue International*, 58:320–25.

46. Calvo, M. S., and Y. K. Park. 1996. Changing phosphorus content of the U.S. diet: Potential for adverse affects on bone. *The Journal Nutrition*, 126:1168s–80s.

47. New, S. A., C. Bolton-Smith, D. A. Grub, and D. M. Reid. 1997. Nutritional influences on bond mineral density: A sectional study in Freeman causal women. *American Journal of Clinical Nutrition*, 65:1831–39.

48. Toss, G. 1992. Effect of calcium intake vs. other lifestyle factors on bone mass. *Journal of Internal Medicine*, 231:181–86.

49. Hoover, P. A. et al. 1996. Postmenopausal bone mineral density: Relationship to calcium intake, calcium absorption, residual estrogen, body

composition, and physical activity. *Canadian Journal of Pharmacology*, 74:911–17.

50. Heaney, R. P., and R. R. Recker. 1986. Distribution of calcium absorption in middle-aged women. *American Journal of Clinical Nutrition*, 43:299–305.

51. Orr-Walker, B. J. et al. 1997. Premature hair graying and bone mineral density. *Journal of Clinical Endocrinology and Metabolism*, 82:3580–83.

52. Michelson, D. et al. 1996. Bone mineral density in women with depression. *New England Journal of Medicine*, 335:1176–81.

53. Seeman, E. 1997. Osteoporosis: Trials and relations. *The American Journal of Medicine*, three (2A):74s–87s.

54. Hoover, P. A. et al.

55. Wats, Nelson B. 1997. Osteoporosis: Prevention, Detection, and Treatment. *Journal of The Medical Association of Georgia*, 86: 224–26.

56. Greenspan, S. L. et al. 1997. Precision and discriminatory ability of the calcaneal bone assessment technologies. *Journal of Bone and Mineral Research*, 12(8):1303–12.

57. Postmenopausal Women. *Calcified Tissue Internationa*l, 60:261–64.

58. Registered trademark of Novartis Pharmaceuticals Corporation.

59. Marchigiano, Gail. 1997. Osteoporosis: Primary prevention and intervention strategies for women at risk. *Own Care Provider*, 2(2):76–83.

60. Registered trademark of Merck & Co., Inc.

61. Registered trademark of Procter & Gamble Pharmaceuticals, Inc., Norwich, NY.

62. Registered trademark of Novartis Pharmaceuticals Corporation.

63. Registered trademark of Procter & Gamble Pharmaceuticals, Corporation.

24 Cancer

1. American Cancer Society. 1992. *Cancer Facts & Figures—1992.* Atlanta: American Cancer Society, Inc., 18–20.

2. Landis, S. et al. 1999. Cancer Statistics, 1999. *A Cancer Journal for Clinicians*, 49 (1).

3. Patterson, R. E. et al. 1997. Vitamin supplements and cancer risk: The epidemiologic evidence. *Cancer Causes and Control*, 8:786–802.

4. Yong, L. et al. 1997. Intake of vitamins B, C, and A and risk of lung cancer. *American Journal of Epidemiology*, 146(3):231–43.

5. Ocke, M. C. et al. 1997. Repeated measurements of vegetables, fruits, beta-carotene, and vitamins C and E in relation to lung cancer. *American Journal of Epidemiology*, 145(4):358–65.

6. Comstock, G. W. 1997. The risk of developing lung cancer associated with antioxidants in the blood: Ascorbic acid, cartenoids, alpha-tocopherol, selenium, and total peroxyl radical absorbing capacity. *Epidemiology, Biomarkers & Prevention*, 6:907–16.

7. Giuliano, A. R. 1997. Antioxidant nutrients: Associations with persistent human papillomavirus infection. *Cancer Epidemiology, Biomarkers & Prevention*, 6:917–23.

8. Grimble, R. F. 1997. Effects of antioxidative vitamins on immune function with clinical applications. *Internat J Vit Nutr*, 67:312–20.

9. Goodman, Marc T. 1997. Association of soy and fiber consumption with the risk of endometrial cancer, *American Journal of Epidemiology*, 146(4):294–306.

10. 1993. Zeroing in on a breast cancer susceptibility gene. *Science*, 259:622–23.

11. Alberg, A .J., and K. J. Helzlsouer. 1997. Epidemiology, prevention, and early detection of breast cancer. *Current Opinion in Oncology*, 9:505–11.

12. Stratton, J. F. et al. 1997. Contributions of BRCA 1 mutations to ovarian cancer. *New England Journal of Medicine*, 336:1125–30.

13. National Alliance of Breast Cancer Organizations. 1998. The diet-breast cancer link. *NABCO News* II(2):1–2.

14. 1993. Focus on Breast cancer: Variety of foods being studied as breast cancer preventatives. *Oncology News International*, (September):22–23.

15. *NABCO News*, 1–2.

16. Boyd, N. P. et al. 1997. Effects at two years of a low-fat, high-carbohydrates diet on radiologic features of the breast: Results from a randomized trial. *Journal of the National Cancer Institute*, 89(7):488–96.

17. Marshall, E. 1993. Search for a killer: Focus shifts from fat to hormones. *Science*, 259:618–21.

18. *NABCO News*, 1–2.

19. Enig, M. G. 1993. Trans fatty acids—an update. *Nutrition Quarterly*, 17(4):79–95.

20. Kohlmeier, L. 1997. Adipose tissue and trans fatty acids and breast cancer in the european community multicenter study on antioxidants, myocardial infarction, and breast cancer. *Cancer Epidemiology, Biomarkers & Prevention*, 6:705–10.

21. Greenwald, Peter, Karen Sherwood, and Sharon S. Mcdonald. 1997. Fat, caloric intake, and obesity: Lifestyle risk factors breasts cancer. *Journal Americans Diet Association*, 97:24–30.

22. Marshall.

23. Marshall.

24. Zeigler, J. April 1992. The dilemma of estrogen replacement therapy. *American Health*. 68–71.
25. Soffa, Virginia M. 1996. Alternatives to hormone replacement for menopause. *Alternative Therapies*, 2(2):34–39.
26. Marshall.
27. Bass, K. M., and T. L. Bush. 1991. Estrogen therapy and cardiovascular risk in women. *Journal of the Louisiana State Medical Society*, 143:33–39.
28. Isenbarger, D. W., and B. I. Chapin. 1997. Current pharmacologic options for prevention and treatment. *Osteoporosis*, 101(1):129–42.
29. Cahn, M. D. et al. 1997. Hormone replacement therapy and the risk of breast lesions that predispose to cancer. *The American Surgeon*, 63:858–60.
30. Veer, P. et. al. 1996. Tissue antioxidants and postmenopausal breast cancer: The European community multicentre study on antioxidants, myocardial infarction, and cancer of the breast. *Cancer Epidemiology, Biomarkers & Prevention*, 5:441–46.
31. Verhoeven, D. T. H. et al. 1997. Vitamins C and E, retinol, beta-carotene and dietary fiber in relation to breast cancer risk: A perspective cohort study. *British Journal of Cancer*, 75(1):149–55.
32. Kushi, L. H. et al. 1996. Intake of vitamins A, C and E and postmenopausal breast cancer. *American Journal of Epidemiology*, 144(2):165–74.
33. van t'Veer, P. et al. 1996. Tissue antioxidants and postmenopausal breast cancer: The European community multicenter study on antioxidants, myocardial infarction, and cancer of the breast (EURAMIC). *Cancer Epidemiology, Biomarkers & Prevention*, 5:441–46.
34. Huang, Z. 1997. Dual effects of weight gain on breast cancer risk. *Journal of the American Medical Association*, 278:1407–11.
35. Wolff, M. S., and A. Weston. 1997. Breast cancer risk and environmental exposures. *Environmental Health Perspectives*, 105(4):891–95.
36. Willett, W. C. 1997. Nutrition and cancer. *Salud Publica de Mexico*, 39(4):298–308.
37. Stoll, B. A. 1997. Micronutrient supplements may reduce breast cancer risk: How, when and which? *European Journal of Clinical Nutrition*, 51:573–77.
38. Nicholson, A. 1996. Diet and the prevention and treatment of breast cancer. *Alternative Therapies*, 2(6):32–38.
39. AHNY. 1997. Diets and stomach cancer in Korea. *International Journal Cancer*, 10:7–9.

40. Lemon, H. M., and J. F. Rodriguez-Sierra. 1996. Timing of breast cancer surgery during the luteal menstrual phase may improve prognosis. *Nebraska Medical Journal*, April:110–15.

41. Biffi, L. et, al. 1997. Antiproliferative effect of fermented milk on the growth of a human breast cancer cell line. *Nutrition and Cancer*, 28(1):93–99.

25 Estrogen and Hormone Replacement Therapy

1. Taylor, Maida. 1997. Alternatives to conventional hormone replacement therapy. *Comprehensive Therapy*, 23(8):514–32.

2. Kessel, Bruce. 1998. Alternatives to estrogen for menopausal women. *Proceedings of the Society for Experimental Biology and Medicine*, 217:38–44.

3. Wolfe, 192–222.

4. Grady, D. et al. 1992. Hormone therapy to prevent disease and prolong life in postmenopausal women. *Annals of Internal Medicine*, 117(12):1016–37.

5. Ibid., 1027–37.

6. Rovner, S. 1989. Estrogen therapy: Boon or risk factor? Women's Health. *Washington Post*, August 8, 1989.

7. National Women's Health Network. 1993. Taking hormones and women's health: Choices, risks and benefits. Washington, D.C.

8. Sotelo, M. M., and S. R. Johnson. 1997. The effects of hormone replacement therapy on coronary heart disease. *Endocrinology and Metabolism Clinics of North America*, 26(2):313–29.

9. Registered trademark of Wyeth-Ayerst Laboratories.

10. Food and Drug Administration. 1990. How to take your estrogen. U.S. Printing Office, (FDA) 91–3186.

11. 1994. *Physicians' Desk Reference*. Montvale, N.J.: Medical Economics Data Production, 2594.

12. Notes from Katherine O'Hanlan, M.D. written in December 1993. Dr. O'Hanlan is an author and physician at Stanford Medical Hospital.

13. Rozenberg, S. et al. 1997. Factors influencing the prescription of hormone replacement therapy. *Obstetrics & Gynecology*, (3):387–91.

14. Komulainen, M. et al. 1997. Vitamin D and HRT: No benefit additional to that of HRT alone in prevention of bone loss in early postmenopausal women. A 2.5-year randomized placebo-controlled study. *Osteoporosis International*, 7:126–32.

15. Barbach, Lonnie. 1993. The Pause. New York: A Dutton Book, 181–82.
16. Persson, I. et al. 1997. Hormone replacement therapy and the risk of breast cancer nested case-control study in a cohort of swedish women attending mammography screening. *International Journal Cancer*, 72:758–61.
17. Cahn, M. D. et al. 1997. Hormone replacement therapy and the risk of breast lesions that predispose to cancer. *The American Surgeon*, 63:858–60.
18. Ibid., 105.
19. Perry, S., and K. O'Hanlan. 1992. *Natural Menopause*. Reading: Addison-Wesley, 86–87.
20. Bass, K. M., and T. L. Bush. 1991. Estrogen therapy and cardiovascular risk in women. *Journal*, 143:33–39.
21. Notes from Katherine O'Hanlan, M.D., in December 1993.
22. Lictman, R. 1991. Perimenopausal hormone replacement therapy: Review of the literature. *Journal of Nurse-Midwifery*, 1:30–48.

26 Exercise

1. Wolfe, S. M. 1991. *Women's health alert*. Reading: Addison-Wesley, 211.
2. Evans, W. J. 1992. Exercise, nutrition and aging. *American Institute of Nutrition*, 122:796–801.
3. American Heart Association. 1993. *Exercise and your heart a guide to physical activity*. Dallas: National Center, 1–37.
4. Sopko, G., E. Obarzanek, and E. Stone. 1992. Overview of the national heart, lung, and blood institute workshop on physical activity and cardiovascular health. *Medicine and Science in Sports and Exercise*, 24(6):192–95.
5. American Heart Association. 1993–1996. *Exercise Diary*. Dallas: National Center. 51-1060.
6. Ibid.
7. Dubois et al. 1992. Moving for health. *Ourselves, growing older*. The Boston Women's Health Book Collective. New York: Simon and Schuster, 62–75.
8. Perry, S., and K. O'Hanlan. 1992. Natural menopause. Reading: Addison-Wesley, 91–93.
9. Kegel, A. M. 1951. Physiologic therapy for urinary stress incontinence. *Journal of the American Medical Association*, 146:915–17.
10. Perry, S., and K. O'Hanlan.

11. Dubois et al.
12. 1997. More ways to stay dry. *Harvard Women's Health Watch*. V(7),2–3.
13. Probart, C. K., P. J. Bird, and K. A. Parker. 1993. Diet and athletic performance. *Clinical Nutrition*, 77(4):757–72.
14. Clarkson, P. M. 1991. Minerals: Exercise performance and supplementation in athletes. *Journal of Sports Science*, 9:91–116.
15. Ibid.
16. Haymes, E. M., and J. J. Lamanca. 1989. Iron loss in runners during exercise: Implications and recommendations. *Sports Medicine*, 7:277–85.
17. Couzy, F., P. Lafargue, and C. Y. Guezennec. 1990. Zinc metabolism in the athlete: Influence of training, nutrition and other factors. *International Journal of Sports Medicine*, 11:263–66.
18. Kanter, M. M., L. A. Nolte, and J. O. Holloszy. 1993. Effects of an antioxidant vitamin mixture on lipid peroxidation at rest and postexercise. *Journal of Applied Physiology*, 74(2):965–69.
19. Goldfarb, A. H. 1993. Antioxidants: Role of supplementation to prevent exercise-induced oxidative stress. *Medicine and Science in Sports and Exercise*, 25(2):232–36.
20. Coyle, E. F. 1991. Timing and method of increased carbohydrate intake to cope with heavy training, competition and recovery. *Journal of Sports Science*, 9:29–52.
21. Evans, W. J. et al. 1983. Protein metabolism and endurance exercise. *Physician and Sportsmedicine*, 11(7):63–72.
22. Lemon, P. W. R. 1991. Effect of exercise on protein requirements. *Journal of Sports Science*, 9:53–70.
23. Position of the American Dietetic Association and the Canadian Dietetic Association. 1993. Nutrition for physical fitness and athletic performance for adults. *Journal of the American Dietetic Association*, 93(6):691–96.
24. Dekkers, C. et al. 1996. The roles of antioxidant vitamins and enzymes in the prevention of exercise-induced muscle damage. *Sports Medicine*, 21(3):213–38.
25. Probart, C. K. et al.
26. Belco, A. Z. et al. 1992. Effects of exercise on riboflavin requirements of young women. *American Jounal of Clinical Nutrition*, 35:783–808.
27. Van Der Beek, E. J. 1991. Vitamin supplementation and physical exercise performance. *Journal of Sports Science*, 9:77–89.
28. Ibid.

29. Simon-Schnass, I., and H. Pabst. 1988. Influence of vitamin E on physical performance. *International Journal of Vitamin and Nutrition Research*, 33:49–54.

30. Madden, M. et al. 1993. Protective effect of vitamin E on exercise-induced oxidative damage in young and older adults. *American Journal of Physiology*, 33:R992–98.

31. Evans.

32. Haymes, E. M., and J. J. Lamanca.

33. Probart, C. K. et al.

34. Couzy, F., P. Lafargue, and C. Y. Guezennec.

35. Economos, C.D., S. S. Bortz, and M. E. Nelson. 1993. Nutritional practices of elite athletes. *Sports Medicine*, 16(6):381–99.

36. Probart, C. K. et al.

37. Position of the American Dietetic Association and the Canadian Dietetic Association.

27 Fish Oils

1. Sanders, T. A. B. 1987. Fish and coronary artery disease. *British Heart Journal*, 57:214–19.

2. Fox, P. L., and P. E. DiCorleto. 1988. Fish oils inhibit endothelial cell production of platelet-derived growth factor-like protein. *Science*, 241:453–56.

3. Dehmer, G. J. et al. 1988. Reduction in the rate of early restenosis after coronary angioplasty by a diet supplemented with n-3 fatty acids. *New England Journal of Medicine*, 319(12):733–40.

4. Levine, P. H. et al. 1989. Dietary supplementation with omega-3 fatty acids prolongs platelet survival in hyperlipidemic patients with atherosclerosis. *Archives of Internal Medicine*, 149:1113–16.

5. Knapp, H. R., and G. A. FitzGerald. 1989. The antihypertensive effects of fish oil. *New England Journal of Medicine*, 320(16):1037–43.

6. Morris, M. C., F. Sacks, and B. Rosner. 1993. Does fish oil lower blood pressure? A meta-analysis of controlled trials. *Circulation*, 88:523–33.

7. Abbey, M., P. Clifton, M. Kestin, B. Belling, and P. Nestel. 1990. Effect of fish oil on lipoproteins, lecithin: Cholesterol acyltransferase, and lipid transfer protein activity in humans. *Arteriosclerosis*, 10:85–94.

8. Kromhout, D. et al. 1985. The inverse relation between fish consumption and 20-year mortality from coronary heart disease. *New England Journal of Medicine*, 312(19):1205–09.

9. Daviglus, M. L. et al. 1997. Fish consumption and the 30-year risk of fatal myocardial infarction. *New England Journal of Medicine*, 336:1046–53.

10. Opstvedt, J. 1997. Fish lipids: More than n-3 fatty acids? *Medical Hypotheses*, 48:481–83.

11. 1996. Increasing fish oil intake—any net benefits? *BNF*, 34(8):60–62.

12. Goode, G. K., S. Garcia, and A. M. Heagerty. 1997. Dietary supplementation with marine fish oil improves in vitro small artery endothelial function in hypercholesterolemic patients. *Circulation*, 96:2802–07.

13. Morcos, N. C. 1997. Modulation of lipid profile by fish oil and garlic combination. *Journal of the National Medical Association*, 89:673–78.

14. Sanders, T. A. B. 1993. Marine oils: Metabolic effects and role in human nutrition. *Proceedings of the Nutrition Society*, 52:457–72.

28 Food

1. Sacks, F. M. et al. 1995. Rationale and design of the dietary approaches to stop hypertension trial (DASH): A multi-center controlled-feeding study of dietary patterns to lower blood pressure. Annals of Epidemiology, 5:108–18.

2. Lawrence J. et al. 1997. A clinical trial of the effects of dietary patterns on blood pressure. *New England Journal of Medicine*, 336:1117.

3. National Heart, Lung and blood Institute. National Institute of Health.

4. National Cancer Institute. 1995. Action guide for healthy eating. NIH Publication No. 95-3877.

5. American Institute for Cancer Research. 1998. Menus and recipes to lower cancer risk. Washington, D.C..

6. The American Heart Association Diet. 1991–1996. *An eating plan for healthy americans.* Dallas: American Heart Association, 2000.

7. Ibid.

8. American Cancer Society. 1996. *Nutrition and cancer prevention.* Atlanta: National Headquarters, 2021-CC.

9. U.S. Department of Agriculture and U.S. Department of Health and Human Services. December 1995. Nutrition and your health: Dietary guidelines for americans. Home and Garden Bulletin No. 232:25 and 9.

10. 1997. *Take charge! A woman's guide to fighting heart disease.* Dallas: The American Heart Association, 64-1055.

11. Ibid.

12. Ibid.

13. Cutler, B. W., and C. Garcia. 1992. *Menopause*. New York: W. W. Norton, 254.
14. National Research Council. 1989. *Recommended dietary allowances*. Washington, D.C.: National Academy Press, 66.
15. Toss, G. 1992. Effect of calcium intake vs. other lifestyle factors on bone mass. *Journal of Internal Medicine*, 231:181–86.
16. Bobroff, L. B. 1988. *Sugar and other sweeteners*. Gainsville: Florida Cooperative Extension Service, University of Florida, 1–6.
17. Perry, S., and K. O'Hanlan. 1992. *Natural Menopause*. Reading: Addison-Wesley, 126–69.
18. Ibid., 128.
19. Blumenthal, D. 1989. *Complex carbohydrates*. Rockville: Department of Health and Human Services, FDA No. 90-2230.
20. Bobroff, L. B. 1988. *Fiber*. Gainesville: Florida Cooperative Extension Service, University of Florida.
21. Hallfrisch, J. et al. 1987. Mineral balances of men and women consuming high fiber diets with complex or simple carbohydrates. *Journal of Nutrition*, 117:48–55.
22. Bobroff, L. B. 1988. *Fats*. Gainesville: Florida Cooperative Extension Service, University of Florida.
23. Kohleier, Lenore. 1997. Biomarkers of fatty acid exposure and breast cancer risk. *American Journal Clinical Nutrition*, 66:1548s–56s.
24. Kuller, Lewis, H. 1997. Dietary fat and chronic diseases: Epidemiology overview. *Journal America in Diet Association*, 97:9–15.
25. Capone, Stefani L., Dilbert Bragga, and John A. Glaspy. 1997. Relationship between omega-3 and omega-6 fatty acid ratios and breast cancer. *In Nutrition*, 13(9).
26. Kohlmeier, Lenore. 1997. Biomarkers of fatty acid exposure and breast cancer risk. *American Journal of Clinical Nutrition*, 66:1548s–56s.
27. Kuller, Lewis, H. 1997. Dietary fat and chronic diseases: Epidemiology overview. *Journal America in Diet Association*, 97:9–15.
28. Enig, M. G., J. Munn, and M. Keeney. 1978. Dietary fat and cancer trends—a critique. *Federation Proceedings*, 37:2215–22.
29. Ibid.
30. Khosla, Pramod, and K. C. Hayes. 1996. Dietary trans-monounsaturated fatty acids negatively impact plasma lipids in humans: Critical review of the evidence. *Journal of the American College of Nutrition*, 15(4):325–39.
31. Willett, W. C. 1994. Diet and health: What should we eat? *Science*, 264:532–37.

32. Enig, M. G. 1993. Trans-fatty acids—an update. *Nutrition Quarterly*, 17(4):79–95.

33. Willett, W. C. et al. 1993. Intake of trans-fatty acids and risk of coronary heart disease among women. *Lancet*, 341:581–85.

34. Enig, M. G. Trans-fatty acids—an update.

35. Kohlmeier, Lenore et al. 1997. Adipose tissue trans-fatty acids and breast cancer in the European community multicenter study on antioxidants, myocardial infarction, and breast cancer. *Cancer Epidemiology, Biomarkers & Prevention*, 6:705–10.

36. Ascherio, A., and W. C. Willett. 1997. Health effects of trans-fatty acids. *American Journal of Clinical Nutrition*, 66(4 Suppl):1006S–1010S.

37. Willett, W. C., and A. Ascherio. 1994. Trans-fatty acids: Are the effects only marginal? *American Journal of Public Health*, 84(5):722–24.

38. Ibid.

39. School of Public Health. September 1993. The new thinking about fats. *University of California Berkeley Wellness Letter*.

40. Schlagheck, Thomas G. et al. 1997. Olestra dose response on fat-soluble nutrients in humans. *Journal Nutrition*, 127:1646s–65s.

41. March 1998. Snack attack olestra. Nutrition Action Health Letter.

42. Procter & Gamble. Final report: Assessment of the dose-response effect of olestra on the status of fat-soluble vitamins and other marker nutrients in humans. Submitted by Procter & Gamble to the FDA on January 29, 1993.

43. Procter & Gamble. An eight-week vitamin restoration study and humans consuming olestra. Submitted by Procter & Gamble to the FDA on June 2, 1993.

44. 1995. *American Journal Clinical Nutrition*, 62:591.

45. Bobroff, L. B. 1988. *Sodium*. Gainesville: Florida Cooperative Extension Service, University of Florida, 1–6.

46. The American Heart Association. 1996. *Sodium and blood pressure*. Dallas: National Center, 50–1092.

47. Stein, P. P., and H. R. Black. 1993. The role of diet in the treatment of hypertension. *Clinical Nutrition*, 77(4):831–47.

48. Ibid., 134–36.

49. Mindell, E. 1985. *Earl Mindell's vitamin bible*. New York: Warner Books, 34, 225.

50. Ibid., 145–46.

51. Upton, G. V. 1990. Lipids, cardiovascular disease, and oral contraceptives: A practical perspective. *Fertility and Sterility*, 53(1):1–12.

52. Perry, 144.

53. Somer, E. 1993. *Nutrition for women*. New York: Henry Holt, 232–34.
54. Walsh, Geoffrey P. 1997. Tea and heart disease. *The Lancet*, 349:735.
55. Ren, Shujun, and Eric J. Lien. 1997. Natural Products and their derivatives as cancer chemopreventive agents. *Progress in Drug Reserve*, 171.

29 The Female Heart

1. 1997. *Take charge! A women's guide to fighting heart disease.* Dallas: The American Heart Association, 64–1055.
2. Bass, K. M., and T. L. Bush. 1991. Estrogen therapy and cardiovascular risk in women. *Journal*, 143:33–39.
3. Utian, W. H., and R. S. Jacobowitz. 1990. *Managing your menopause.* New York: Prentice Hall Press, 38–39.
4. Sopko, G., E. Obarzanek, and E. Stone. 1992. Overview of the national heart, lung, and blood institute workshop on physical activity and cardiovascular health. *Medicine and Science in Sports and Exercise*, 24(6):192–95.
5. Barrett, C. C., M. Kirtley, and R. Mangham. 1991. Mitral valve prolapse. *Journal of the Louisiana State Medical Society*. 143(5):41–43.
6. Wilcken, D. E. 1992. Genes, gender and geometry and the prolapsing mitral valve. *Australian and New Zealand Journal of Public Health Medicine*, 22(5 suppl):556–61.
7. Devereux, R. B. 1995. Recent developments in the diagnosis and management of mitral valve prolapse. *Current Opinion in Cardiology*, 10(2):107–16.
8. 1997. Take Charge! A women's guide to fighting heart disease. Dallas: The American Heart Association, 64–1055.
9. Ibid.
10. Willett, W. C. 1994. Diet and health: What should we eat? *Science*, 264:532–37.
11. Schwartz, Steven M. et al. 1997. Myocardial infarction in young women in relation to plasma total homocysteine, folate, and a common variant in the methylenetetrahydrofolate reductase gene. *Circulation*, 96:412–17.
12. Shimakawa, T. et al. 1997. Vitamin intake: A possible determinant of plasma homocysteine among the middle-aged adults. *Annals of Epidemiology*, 7:285–93.
13. Lussier-CaCan, S. et al. 1996. Plasma total homocysteine in healthy subjects: Sex-specific relation with biological trait. *American Journal of Clinical Nutrition*, 64:587-93.

14. Brattstrom, Lars. 1996. Vitamins as homocysteine-lowering agents. *Journal of Nutrition*, 126:1276–80.

15. Parnetti, L., T. Bottiglieri, and D. Lowenthaw. 1997. Role of Homocysteine in age-related vascular and non-vascular diseases. *Alcoholism, Clinical, and Experimental Research*, 9:241–57.

16. Frans, P. V. et. al. 1997. Plasma total homocysteine, B vitamins, and risk of coronary atherosclerosis. *Arteriosclerosis, Thrombosis, and Vascular Biology*, 17:989–95.

17. Duell, P. B., and R. Malinow. 1997. Homocysteine: An important risk factor for atherosclerotic and vascular disease. *Current Opinion in Lipidology*, 8:28–34.

18. Welch, G. N. et al. 1997. Homocysteine, oxidative stress, and vascular disease. *Hospital Practice*, (June 15):81–92.

19. Cook, P. J. et al. 1998. Chlamydia pneumonia antibody titers are significantly associated with acute stroke and transient cerebral ischemia: The West Birmingham stroke project. *Stroke*, 29(2):404–10.

20. Meniconi, A. G., and T. F. Luscher. 1998. Is arteriosclerosis an infectious disease? *Schwizerische Rundschau for Medizin Praxis*, 87(3):64–74.

21. Ottesen, B., and M. B. Sorensen. 1997. Women at cardiac risk: Is HRT the route to maintaining cardiovascular health? *International Journal of Gynecology & Obstetrics*, 59(1), 19–27.

30 Herbs

1. Kaldas, R. S., and C. L. Hughes. 1989. Reproductive and general metabolic effects of phytoestrogens in mammals. *Reproductive Toxicology*, 3:81–89.

2. Murray, M., and J. Pizzorno. 1991. *Encyclopedia of natural medicine*. Rockland: Prima Publishing, 461–62.

3. Gavaler, J. S. 1993. Alcohol and nutrition in postmenopausal women. *Journal of the American College of Nutrition*, 12(4):349–56.

4. Fenwick, G. R., and A. B. Hanley. 1985. The genus allium—Part 3. *CRC Critical Reviews in Food Science and Nutrition*, 23(1):1–73.

5. Fogarty, M. 1993. Garlic's potential role in reducing heart disease. *BJCP*, 47(2):64–65.

6. Fenwick, G. R., and A. B. Hanley.

7. Warshafsky, S., R. S. Kramer, and S. L. Sivak. 1993. Effect of garlic on total serum cholesterol: A meta-analysis. *Annals of Internal Medicine*, 119:599–605.

8. Kiesewetter, H. et al. 1991. Effect of garlic on thrombocyte aggregation, microcirculation, and other risk factors. *International Journal of Clinical Pharmacology Therapy and Toxicology*, 29(4):151–55.

9. Steinmetz, K. A. et al. 1994. Vegetables, fruit and colon cancer in the Iowa Women's Health Study. *American Journal of Epidemiology*, 139:(1)1–15.

10. Han, J. 1993. Highlights of the cancer chemoprevention studies in China. *Prevention Medicine*, 22:712–22.

11. Farber, K. S., E. D. Barnett, and G. R. Bolduc. 1993. Antibacterial activity of garlic and onions: A historical perspective. *Pediatric Infectious Disease Journal*, 12(7):613–14.

12. Elghamry, M. I., and I. M. Shihata. 1966. Biological activity of phytoestrogens. *Veterinary Medicine*, Cairo University, UAR, 352–57.

13. Murray, M., and J. Pizzorno.

14. Messina, M., and S. Barnes. 1991. The role of soy products in reducing risk of cancer. *Journal of National Cancer Research*, 83(8):541–46.

15. National Cancer Institute. 1998. Cancer trials.

16. Murray, M., and J. Pizzorno.

17. Messina, Mark, Stephen Barnes, and Kenneth D. Satchel. 1997. Photoestrogen end rest cancer. *The Lancet*, 350:971–72.

18. Knight, David C., and John A. Eden. 1996. A Review of the clinical effects of phytoestrogens. *Obstetrics & Gynecology*, 87(5):897–904.

19. Ren, Shujun, and Eric J. Lien. 1997. Natural products and their derivatives as cancer chemopreventive agents. *Progress in Drug Reserve*, 171.

20. Nagata, C. et al. 1998. Decreased serum cholesterol concentration is associated with high intake of soy products in Japanese men and women. *Journal of Nutrition*, 128:203–13.

21. Kurzer, Mindy S., and Xia Xu. 1997. Dietary phytoestrogens. *Annual Review of Nutrition*, 17:353–81.

22. Messina, M., and S. Barnes.

23. Aldercreutz, H. et al. 1991. Urinary excretion of lignans and isoflavonoid phytoestrogens in Japanese men and women consuming a traditional Japanese diet. *American Journal of Clinical Nutrition*, 54:1093–100.

24. Fukutake, M. et al. 1996. Quantification of genistein and genistin in soybeans and soybean products. *Food and Chemical Toxicology*, 34:457–61.

25. Michnovicz, Jon J. 1996. Plant estrogens and human and health. *Annals of Surgical Oncology*, 3(6):513–14.

26. Zava, D. T., M. Blen, and G. Duwe. 1997. Estrogenic activity of natural and synthetic estrogens in human breast cancer cells in culture. *Environmental health perspectives*, 105(3):637–45.

27. Hopkins, M. P., L. Androff, and A. S. Benninghoff. 1988. Ginseng face cream and unexplained vaginal bleeding. *American Journal of Obstetrics and Gynecology*, 159(5):1121–22.

28. Petrakis, N. L. et al. 1996. Stimulatory influence of soy protein isolate on the breast secretion in pre- and postmenopausal women. *Cancer Epidemiology, Biomarkers & Prevention*, 5:785–94.

29. Bennetts, H. W., E. J. Underwood, and F. L. Shier. 1946. A specific breeding problem of sheep on subterranean clover pastures in western Australia. *Australian Veterinary Journal*, 22:2–12.

30. Setchell, K. D. R. et al. 1987. Dietary estrogens—a probable cause of infertility and liver disease in captive cheetahs. *Gastroenterology*, 93:225–33.

31. Okwuasaba, F. K. et al. 1991. Anticonceptive and estrogenic effects of a seed extract of *Ricinus communis* var. *minor*. *Journal of Ethnopharmacology*, 34:141–45.

32. Vessal, M., H. A. Mehrani, and G. H. Omrani. 1991. Effects of an aqueous extract of Physalis alkekengi fruit on estrus cycle, reproduction and uterine creatine kinase BB-isozyme in rats. *Journal of Ethnopharmacology*, 34:69–78.

33. Stoll, B. A. Eating to beat breast cancer: Potential role for soy supplements. Oncology Department, Saints Common Hospital, London's UK.

34. Mirkin, G. 1991. Estrogens in Yams. *Journal of the American Medical Association*, 265(7):912.

35. Zhu, David P. Q. 1987. Dong quai. *American Journal of Chinese Medicine*, xv(3-4):117–25.

36. Hirata, J. D. et al. 1997. Does dong quai have estrogenic effects in postmenopausal women? A double-blind, placebo-controlled trial. *Fertility and Sterility*, 68:981–86.

37. Punnonen, R., and A. Lukola. 1980. Oestrogen-like effect of ginseng. *British Medical Journal*, 281.

38. Marasco, C. A. et al. 1996. Double-blind study of a multivitamin complex supplemented with ginseng extract. *Drugs Under Experimental and Clinical Research*, 22(6):323–29.

39. See, D. M. et al. 1997. In vitro effects of echinacea and ginseng all in natural killer and antibody-dependent cell cytotoxicity in healthy subjects

and chronic fatigue syndrome or acquired immune syndrome patients. *Immunopharmacology*, 35:229–35.

40. Vaya, J. et al. 1997. Antioxidant constituents from licorice roots: Isolation, structure elucidation and antioxidant capacity for LDL oxidation. *Free Radical Biology & Medicine*, 23(2):302–13.

41. Albert-Puleo, M. 1980. Fennel and anise as estrogenic agents. *Journal of Ethnopharmacology*, 2:337–44.

42. Zondek, B., and E. Bergmann. 1938. LXXXIV. Phenol methyl ethers as oestrogenic agents. *Biochemistry*, XXXII:41–645.

43. Smith, P. F., K. Maclennan, and C. L. Darlington. 1996. The neuroprotective properties of the ginkgo biloba leaf: A review of the possible relationship to platelet-activating factor. *Journal of Ethnopharmacology*, 50:131–39.

44. Petkov, V. D. 1993. Memory effects of standardize extracts of panax and ginseng (G115) Ginkgo Biloba (GK 501) and their combination gincosan® (PHL-00701). *Planta Medica*, 59:106–14.

45. Kanowski, S. et al. 1996. Proof of efficacy of the ginkgo biloba special extract EGb a761 in outpatients suffering from mild to moderate primary degenerative dementia of the alzheimer type or multi-infarct dementia. *Pharmacopsychiatry*, 29:47–56.

46. Valenti, G. 1997. DHEA replacement therapy for human aging: A call for perspective. *Alcoholism, Clinical, and Experimental Research*, 9(4):71–72.

47. Evans, Michael F., and Katie Morganster. 1997. St. John's wort: An herbal remedy for depression? *Canadian Family Physicians*, 48:1735–36.

31 Menopause

1. Budoff, P. W. 1984. *No more hot flashes*. New York: Warner Books, 3–9.

2. Perry, S., and K. O'Hanlan. 1992. *Natural menopause*. Reading: Addison-Wesley, 17.

3. Ibid., 9.

4. Utian, W. H., and R. S. Jacobowitz. 1990. *Managing your menopause*. New York: Prentice Hall, 35.

5. Perry, 90.

6. Sheehy, G. 1992. *Silent passages*. New York: Random House, 23.

7. Perry, S., and K. O'Hanlan. 28–35.

8. Weber, G. 1990. A season for sex. *Health/sharing*, Fall/winter 18–21.

9. Perry, S. and K. O'Hanlan. 84–87.

10. Soffa, Virginia M. 1996. Alternatives to hormone replacement for menopause. *Alternative Therapies*, 2(2):34–39.
11. Shaw, Christine. 1997. The perimenopausal hot flash: Epidemiology, physiology, and treatments. *The Nurse Practitioners*, 2(3):55–65.
12. Albrecht, A. E. et al. 1996. Effect of estrogen replacement therapy on natural killer cell activity in postmenopausal women. *Maturitas*, 25:217–22.
13. Perry, S., and K. O'Hanlan. 32.
14. Lucero, M. A., and W. W. McCloskey. 1997. Alternatives to estrogen for the treatment of hot flashes. *The Annals of Pharmacology*, 31:915–17.
15. Registered trademark of Eli Lilly & Company.
16. Bryant, H. U., and W. H. Dere. 1998. Selective estrogen receptor modulators: An alternative to hormone replacement therapy. *Proceedings of the Society for Experimental Biology and Medicine*, 217:45–52.
17. Valenti, G. 1997. DHEA replacement therapy for human aging: A call for perspective. *Alcoholism, Clinical and Experimental Research*, 9(4):71–72.
18. Taylor, Maida. 1997. Alternatives to conventional hormone replacement therapy. *Comprehensive Therapy*, 23(8):514–32.
19. Miller, Richard A. 1997. DHEA brass ring or red herring? *Journal of the American Geriatrics Society*, 45(11):1402–03.
20. Yen, S. S. C., A. J. Morales, and O. Khorram. Replacement of DHEA in aging men and women. Department of Reproductive Medicine, University of California, San Diego.
21. Oklahoma Poison Control Center. 1997. DHEA. . . friend or foe? *Journal Oklahoma State Medical Association*, 90(7):412.
22. Whitehead, Malcolm. 1996. Treatments for menopausal and post-menopausal problems: Present and future. *Bailliere's Clinical Obstetrics and Gynecology*, 10(3), 516–31.

32 Premenstraul Syndrome (PMS)

1. Martorano, J., M. Morgan, and W. Fryer. 1993. Unmasking PMS the complete medical treatment plan. New York: M. Evans, 201.
2. Abraham, G. E. 1983. Nutritional factors in the etiology of the premenstrual tension syndromes. *Journal of Reproductive Medicine*, 28(7):446–64.
3. Abraham, G. E., and J. T. Hargrove. 1980. Effect of vitamin B_6 on premenstrual symptomatology in women with premenstrual tension syndromes: A double blind crossover study. *Infertility*, 3(2):155–65.

4. Dalton, K., and M. J. T. Dalton. 1987. Characteristics of pyridoxine overdose neuropathy syndrome. *Acta Neurol Scand*, 76:8–11.

5. Dalton, K. 1984. *The premenstrual syndrome and progesterone therapy*. Chicago: Yearbook Medical Publishers, 124.

6. Martorano, J., M. Morgan, and W. Fryer, 172.

7. Abraham, G. E. 452.

8. Martorano, J., M. Morgan, and W. Fryer, 171.

9. Mindell, E. 1985. *Earl Mindell's vitamin bible*. New York: Warner Books, 235.

10. Maxson, W. S., and J. T. Hargrove. 1985. Bioavailability of oral micronized progesterone. *Fertility and Sterility*, 44(5):622–26.

11. Martorano, J. T., M. Ahlgrimm, and D. Myers. 1993. Differentiating between natural progesterogens: Clinical implications for premenstrual syndrome management. *Comprehensive Therapy*, 19(3):96–98.

12. Martorano, J., M. Morgan, and W. Fryer, 194.

13. Moline, M. L. 1993. Pharmacologic strategies for managing premenstrual syndrome. *Clinical Pharmacology*, 12:181–96.

14. Plouffe, L. et al. 1994. Premenstrual syndrome update on diagnosis and management. *The Female Patient*, 19:53–58.

15. Registered trademark of Eli Lilly & Company.

16. Registered trademark of Pfizer, Inc.

17. Korzekwa, Marilyn I., and Meir Steiner. 1997. Premenstrual syndromes. *Clinical Obstetrics and Gynecology*, (3):564–76.

18. Sundblad, C. et al. 1997. A naturalistic listed study of paroxetine in premenstrual syndrome: Efficacy and side-effects during ten cycles of treatment. *Europeans Neuropsychopharmacology*, 7:201–06.

19. Korzekwa, Marilyn I., and Meir Steiner.

20. Su, T. et al. 1997. Fluoxetine and the treatment of premenstrual dysphoria. *Neuropsychopharmacology*, 16(5):346–56.

33 Skin and Aging

1. Novick, N. L. 1988. *Super Skin*. New York: Clarkson N. Potter, 4.

2. Wyngaarden, J. B., L. H. Smith, and J. C. Bennett. 1992. *Cecil Textbook of Medicine*. Philadelphia: W. B. Saunders, 2282–86.

3. Kurban, R. S., and J. Bhawan. 1990. Histologic changes in skin associated with aging. *Journal of Dermatologic Surgery and Oncology*, 16:909.

4. Ibid., 908–14.

5. Ibid., 911.

6. Ibid., 911.

7. Lavker, R. M., P. Zheng, and G. Dong. 1986. Morphology of aged skin. *Dermatologic Clinics*. Philadelphia: W. B. Saunders, 4(3):379–89.

8. Downing, D. T., M. E. Stewart, and J. S. Strauss. 1986. Changes in sebum secretion and the sebaceous gland. *Dermatologic Clinics*. Philadelphia: W. B. Saunders, 4(3):419–23.

9. Warren, R. et al. 1991. Age, sunlight, and facial skin: A histologic and quantitive study. *Journal of the American Academy of Dermatology*, 25:751–60.

10. Lavker, R. M., P. Zheng, and G. Dong.

11. Sams, W. M. 1986. Sun-induced aging: Clinical and laboratory observations in man. *Dermatologic Clinics*. Philadelphia: W. B. Saunders, 4(3):509–16.

12. Lavker, R. M., P. Zheng, and G. Dong.

13. Pathak, M. A. 1991. Ultraviolet radiation and the development of non-melanoma and melanoma skin cancer: Clinical and experimental evidence. *Skin Pharmacology*, 4(1):85–94.

14. American Cancer Society. 1992. Cancer facts and figures—1992. Alanta: American Cancer Society, Inc., 17–20.

15. Ibid.

16. Perry, S., and K. O'Hanlan. 1992. *Natural menopause*. Reading: Addison-Wesley, 169–70.

17. Burke, K. E. 1990. Facial wrinkles: Prevention and nonsurgical correction. *Postgraduate Medicine*, 88(1):207–28.

18. Registered trademark of Ortho Pharmaceutical Corporation.

19. Registered trademark of Ortho Pharmaceutical Corporation.

20. Registered trade name of Berner Ltd. Finland.

21. Registered trade name of Scandinavian Natural Health and Beauty Products, Inc.

22. Eskelinen, A., and J. Santalhti. 1992. Special natural cartilage polysaccharides for the treatment of sun-damaged skin in females. *Journal of International Medical Research*, 20:99–105.

23. Pinski, K. S., and H. H. Roenigk. 1992. Autologous fat transplantation. *Journal of Dermatologic Surgery and Oncology*, 18:179–84.

24. Novick, N. L., 209–10.

25. Zaias, N. 1990. *The nail in health and disease*. Norwalk: Appleton & Lange, 11, 164.

26. Ibid., 165.

27. Brown, Algie C. Toenail party time with tinea pedis. Microbiology Lecture, American Academy of Dermatology 56th Annual Meeting, Feb. 28, 1998.

28. The registered trademark of Pharmacia and UpJohn.

29. The registered trademark of Merck & Co., Inc.
30. Hendler, S. S. 1990. *The doctor's vitamin and mineral encyclopedia.* New York: Simon and Schuster, 277–78.
31. Klein, A. D., and N. S. Penneys. 1998. Aloe vera. *Journal of the American Academy of Dermatology*, 18:714–20.
32. Olsen, E .A. et al. 1992. Tretinoin emollient cream: A new therapy for photodamaged skin. *Journal of the American Academy of Dermatology*, 26:215–24.
33. Brodell, L. P., D. Asselin, and R. T. Brodell. 1992. Reversible ectropion after long-term use of topical tretinoin on photodamaged skin. *Journal of the American Academy of Dermatology*, 27(4):621–22.
34. David, L. M. 1985. Laser vermillion ablation for actinic cheilitis. *Journal of Dermatologic Surgery and Oncology*, 11:605–08.
35. Dufresne, R. G. Jr. et al. 1988. Carbon dioxide laser treatment of chronic actinic cheilitis. *Journal of the American Academy of Dermatology*, 19:876–78.
36. Whitaker, D. C. 1987. Microscopically proven cure of actinic cheilitis by CO_2 laser. *Lasers Surgery Medicine*, 7:520–23.
37. Registered trademark of Coherent Medical, Palo Alto, CA.
38. Registered trademark of Sharplan Lasers, Inc., Allentown, PA.
39. David, L. M. et al. 1989. CO_2 laser abrasion for cosmetic and therapeutic treatment of facial actinic damage. *Cutis*, 43:583–87.
30. Lask, G. et al. 1995. Laser skin resurfacing with the Silktouch flashscanner for facial rhytides. *Dermatologic Surgery*, 21:1021–24.
41. Lowe, N. et al. 1995. Skin resurfacing with the Ultrapulse carbon dioxide laser. *Dermatologic Surgery*, 21:1025–29.
42. Waldorf, H. A., A. B. Kauvar, and R. G. Geronemus. 1995. Skin resurfacing of fine to deep rhytides using a char-free carbon dioxide laser in 47 patients. *Dermatologic Surgery*, 21:940–46.
43. Trelles, M. A., L. M. David, and J. Rigau. 1996. Penetration depth of Ultrapulse carbon dioxide laser in human skin. *Dermatologic Surgery*, 22:863–65.
44. Kauvar, A. B., H. A. Waldorf, and R. G. Geronemus. 1996. Histological comparison of "charfree" carbon dioxide lasers. *Dermatologic Surgery*, 22:343–48.
45. Ho, C. et al. 1995. Laser resurfacing in pigmented skin. *Dermatologic Surgery*, 21:1035–37.
46. Fitzpatrick, R. E. I. et al. 1996. Pulsed carbon dioxide laser resurfacing of photo-aged facial skin. *Archives of Dermatology*, 132(4):395–402.
47. Ibid.

48. Stuzin, J. M., T. J. Baker, and A. M. Kligman. 1992. Histologic effects of the high energy pulsed CO_2 laser on photo-aged facial skin. *Plastic and Reconstructive Surgery*, Jun,99(7):2036–50.
49. Roberts, T. L., and C. Weinstein. 1995. High energy ultrapulsed CO_2 laser for correction of wrinkles and skin surface irregularities. Abstract presented at American Society for Plastic and Reconstructive Surgery.
50. Trelles, M. A. et al. 1998. A clinical and histological comparison of flashscanning versus pulsed technology in carbon dioxide laser facial skin resurfacing. *Dermatologic Surgery*, 24:43–49.
51. Roberts and Weinstein.
52. Fulton, J. E., and T. Barnes. 1998. Collagen shrinkage (selective dermaplasty) with the high-energy pulsed carbon dioxide laser. *Dermatologic Surgery*, 24:37–41.
53. Stuzin, Baker, and Kligman.
54. Apfelberg, D. B. 1997. A critical appraisal of high-energy pulsed carbon dioxide laser facial resurfacing for acne scars. *Annals of Plastic Surgery*, 99(4):1094–98.
55. Alster, T. S., and T. B. West. 1996. Resurfacing of atrophic facial acne scars with a high-energy, pulsed carbon dioxide laser. *Dermatologic Surgery*, 22:151–55.
56. Lowe, N., G. Lask, and M. Griffin. 1995. Laser skin resurfacing, pre- and posttreatment guidelines. *Dermatologic Surgery*, 21:1017–19.
57. Registered trademark of C. R. Bard Medical Division, Inc. Covington, GA.
58. Registered trademark of Spenco Medical Corp., Waco, TX.
59. Duke, D., and J. M. Grevelink. 1998. Care before and after laser skin resurfacing: A survey and review of the literature. *Dermatologic Surgery*, 24:201–08.
60. Lowe, Lask, and Griffin.
61. Duke and Grevelink.
62. Weinstein, C. Ultrapulse carbon dioxide laser resurfacing presentation to Lahey Hitchcock Clinic Aesthetic Laser Surgery Symposium November 1995.
63. Waldorf, H. A., A. B. Kauvar, and R. G. Geronemus. 1995. Skin resurfacing of fine to deep rhytides using a char-free carbon dioxide laser in 47 patients. *Dermatologic Surgery*, 21:940–46.
64. Weinstein, C., O. Ramirez, and J. Pozner. 1998. Postoperative care following carbon dioxide laser resurfacing. Avoiding pitfalls. *Dermatologic Surgery*, 24:51–56.
65. Weinstein.

66. Lowe, Lask, and Griffin.
67. Duke, and Grevelink.
68. Ibid.
69. Nanni, C., and T. Alster. 1998. Complications of cutaneous laser surgery: A review. *Dermatologic Surgery*, 24:209–20.
70. Trelles, M. A. et al. 1998. The origin and role of erythema after carbon dioxide laser resurfacing: A clinical and histological study. *Dermatologic Surgery*, 24:25–29.
71. Fulton, and Barnes.
72. Trelles, M. A. et al.
73. Kaufmann, R., and R. Hibst. 1996. Pulsed erbium:yag laser ablation in cutaneous surgery. *Laser Surgery*, 19(3):324–30.
74. 1997. Resurfacing of pitted facial scars with a pulsed Er:yag laser. *Dermatology Surgery*, 23(10):880–83.
75. Registered trademark of Sharplan Lasers, Inc., Allentown, PA.
76. Registered trademark of Tissue Technologies, Palomar Medical Products, Inc., Lexington, MA.
77. Kim, J. W., and J. O. Lee. 1997. Skin resurfacing in Asians. *Aesthetic Plastic Surgery*, 21(2):115–17.
78. Nanni, and Alster.
79. Registered trademark of Roche Laboratories, Inc. Nutley, NJ.

34 Weight

1. Jacobowitz, R. S. 1993. *150 most-asked questions about menopause.* New York: Hearst Books, 200.
2. Perry, S., and K. O'Hanlan. 1992. *Natural menopause.* Reading: Addison-Wesley, 122.
3. Lapidus, L. et al. 1986. Dietary habits in relation to incidence of cardiovascular disease and death in women: A 12-year follow-up of participants in the population study of women in Gothenburg, Sweden. *Journal of Clinical Nutrition*, 44:444–48.
4. American Heart Association. *Heart stroke facts.* Dallas: National Headquarters, 38.
5. Hocman, G. 1988. Prevention of cancer: Restriction of nutritional energy intake (joules). *Comparative Biochemistry Physiology*, 91A(2):209–20.
6. American Cancer Association. *Cancer figures and facts—1992.* Atlanta: National Headquarters, 20.

7. Tsukamoto, H., and F. Sano. 1990. Body weight and longevity: Insurance experience in Japan. *Diabetes Research and Clinical Practice*, 10:119–25.

8. Rissanen, A. et al. 1991. Weight and mortality in Finnish women. *Journal of Clinical Epidemiology*, 44(8):787–95.

9. Morley, J. E. 1987. Nutritional problems of the elderly. Bol Asoc Medical Clinic Puerto Rico, 79(12):505–07.

10. Goldstein, D. J. 1992. Beneficial health effects of modest weight loss. *International Journal of Obesity*, 16:397–415.

11. Lee, I., and R. S. Paffenbarger. 1992. Change in body weight and longevity. *Journal of the American Medical Association*, 268:2045–49.

12. Williamson, D. F. 1997. Intentional weight loss: Patterns in the general population and its association with morbidity and mortality. *International Journal of Obesity*, 21(1):14–19.

13. Levy, A. S., and A. W. Heaton. 1993. Weight control practices of U.S. adults trying to lose weight. *Annals of Internal Medicine*, 119(7pt2):661–66.

14. Utian, W. H., and R. S. Jacobowitz. 1990. *Managing your menopause*. New York: Prentice Hall, 101–02.

15. Anderson, R. E., T. A. Wadden, and R. J. Herzog. 1997. Changes in bone mineral content in obese dieting women. *Metabolism*, 46(8):857–61.

16. The National Heart, Lung, and Blood Institute. The National Institute of Health. Information: P.O. Box 30105, Bethesda, Maryland 20824-0105.

17. Monteleone, G., and D. G. Browing. 1997. Nutrition in women. *Primary Care*, 24(1),37–51.

18. Toubro, S. et al. 1993. Safety and efficacy of long-term treatment with ephedrine, caffeine and ephedrine/caffeine mixture. *International Journal of Obesity*, 17(1):69–72.

19. Wiener, P. K., and R. C. Young. 1995. Ephedrine-induced mania from herbal diet supplement. *American Journal Psychiatry*, 152(4):647.

20. Bruno, A., K. B. Nolte, and J. Chapin. 1993. Stroke associated with ephedrine use. *Neurology*, 43:1313–16.

21. Krzanowski, J. J. 1996. Chromium picolinate. *Journal of Florida Medical Association*, 83(1):29–31.

22. Trent, L. K., and D. Thieding-Cancel. 1995. Effects of chromium picolinate on body composition. Journal of Sports Medicine and Physical Fitness, 35:273–80.

23. Leung, L. H. 1995. Pantothenic acid as a weight-reducing agent: Fasting without hunger, weakness end ketosis. *Medical Hypothesis*, 44:403–05.

24. *Managing your weight*, Dallas: American Heart Association, 50-1085.

36 Chiropractic

1. Levin-Gervasi, Stephanie. 1996. *The back pain source book*. Los Angeles, CA: Lowell House, 109.
2. Cherkin, Daniel C. Ph.D., and Robert D. Mootz, DC, ed. Chiropractic in the United States: Training, practice, and research. (Agency for Health Care Policy and Research, Publication No. 98-N002), 7, 2.
3. Cherkin and Mootz, 6.
4. Kandel, Joseph, M.D., and David B. Sudderth, M.D. 1996. *Back pain what works!* Rocklin, CA: Prima Publishing, 110.
5. Langone, John. 1982. *Chiropractors: A consumer's guide*. Reading, MA: Addison-Wesley, 47.
6. Cherkin and Mootz, 4, 1.
7. Ibid., 3, 2.
8. Journal of the American Chiropractic Association. 1997-98 Membership Directory. Arlington, VA: American Chiropractic Association, 34:45.
9. Ibid., 45.
10. American Chiropractic Association. Doctor of chiropractic: Occupational description, #F-21.
11. Cherkin, and Mootz, 11, 6.
12. Ibid., 7, 2.
13. Ibid., 3, 11.
14. Ibid., 3, 11.
15. Ibid., 12, 1.
16. Ibid., 6, 7.

38 Allopathic Medicine

1. Loudon, Irving. 1997. *Oxford Western Medicine*. New York: Oxford University Press.
2. Porter, Roy. 1997. *Medicine a history of healing*. New York: Marlowe.
3. Ritchie, David, and Fred Israel. 1995. Life in America 100 years ago. *Health and medicine*. New York: Chelsea House.

4. U.S. Department of Labor Bureau of Labor Statistics. 1998. *Occupational outlook handbook*. Washington, D.C. Bulletin 2500.

39 Recommendations

1. National Research Council. 1989. Recommended dietary allowances. Washington, D.C.: National Academy Press. 13.

Index

Acid peels for skin rejuvenation, 204–5
Acne, retinoids for, 17, 20, 22
Actinic keratoses, 200
Acupuncture, 225, 231–32. *See also* Traditional Chinese medicine
African-American women
  cancer in, 114
  high blood pressure in, 173
Age spots, 202
Aging skin
  aging's effect on skin, 197–98
  graying hair and hair loss, 34, 109, 208–10
  laser resurfacing for wrinkles, 206, 212–16
  nails, 207–8
  skin cancer, 20, 113, 114, 199, 200–201, 203
  skin nutrients and treatments, 211–12
  smoking and, 199
  spots, keratoses, carcinomas, and moles, 200–202
  sun damage, 198–99
  sun damage prevention and treatment, 202–7
Alcohol, 169
  breast cancer risk and, 119–20
  as calcium antagonist, 69
  chromium in, 72
  as folate antagonist, 32
  as inositol antagonist, 35
  iron absorption and, 80
  in moderation, 169, 261
  N-nitroso compounds in, 39
  as osteoporosis risk factor, 108, 109
  as PABA antagonist, 35
  potassium loss and, 94
  as pyridoxine (B_6) antagonist, 30
  red wine, 175
  retinol and, 19
  riboflavin requirements and, 26
  summary of information on, 169
  as thiamine antagonist, 25
  as vitamin B_{12} antagonist, 33
  as vitamin C antagonist, 41
Alcoholics
  magnesium absorption in, 86
  niacin deficiency (pellagra) in, 27
  thiamine deficiency (Wernicke-Korsakoff syndrome) in, 24
Allopathic (traditional Western) medicine
  Eastern medicine versus, 226–29
  history and description of, 249–52
  integration of Chinese medicine with, 230–32
Aloe vera, 211
Alpha-hydroxy acid moisturizers, 206–7
Alzheimer's disease
  choline for memory loss, 36

estrogen replacement therapy and, 125
ginkgo biloba for, 184
vitamin E for, 47, 51
Amino acids, 158–59
Anemia
iron for, 79
vitamin B_{12} for pernicious anemia, 33
Angiomas, senile, 201
Anise, 183
Anorexia nervosa, bone loss and, 66, 104
Antacids as calcium supplements, 68
Antagonists, defined, 10–11
Antibiotics
as biotin antagonists, 34
as vitamin C antagonists, 41
Antioxidants
for athletes, 135–36
for cancer prevention, 114–15, 118–19
CoQ_{10}, 59–61
free radicals and, 9, 50, 136
green and black tea, 170
selenium, 95–97
vitamin A (beta-carotene), 17–22
vitamin C, 37–42
vitamin E, 47–53
Antistress vitamin, pantothenic acid (B_5) as, 28
Antituberculosis drugs and need for vitamin B_6, 30
Apocrine glands, defined, 197
Atherosclerosis. *See also* Heart disease
beta-carotene for, 17
fish oils for, 147–48
homocysteine levels and, 174–75
Athletic performance
CoQ_{10} for, 59, 60–61
diet and, 135–37
thiamine for, 24, 136
vitamin E for, 50

B vitamins, 23–36
for athletes, 135, 136
choline, 36
cyanocobalamin (B_{12}), 32–33
dosage range, 255–56
folic acid, 30–32
functions of, 23
homocysteine levels and, 174–75
inositol, 35
niacin (B_3), 26–28
pantothenic acid (B_5), 28–29, 221–22
para-aminobenzoic acid (PABA), 34–35, 203
pyridoxine (B_6), 29–30, 192, 193
riboflavin (B_2), 25–26, 136
thiamine (B_1), 24–25, 136
Back Pain: What Works!, 237
Basal cell carcinomas, 199, 200
Bayer aspirin, 251
Beriberi, 7, 24
Beta-carotene (vitamin A)
for breast cancer prevention, 17, 18, 19, 114, 119
defined, 18
food sources of, 20
for lung cancer prevention, 17, 19–20
for mastodynia (sore breasts), 17, 19
olestra and, 117, 165
as protective agent against heart attack, 18
Bioavailability, defined, 10
Bioflavonoids, defined, 40
Biotin
dosage range, 256
for hair, 34, 211
summary of information on, 34
Birth control pills. *See* Oral contraceptives
Birth defects
folic acid for prevention of, 30–31
warning regarding vitamin A and, 22
Black cohosh, 183
Black women
cancer in, 114
high blood pressure in, 173

Bladder control, 133–35, 210
Blood clotting, vitamin K and, 55
Blood pressure, 173–74. *See also* High blood pressure
Blood thinners, warning regarding vitamin K and, 57
Body mass index (BMI) chart, 219–21
Body weight. *See* Weight
Bonemeal, 68
Bones, 103–11. *See also* Osteoporosis; Osteoporosis prevention
  anatomy, 103
  bone mineral density measurement, 110–11
  exercise for good bone mineral density, 106, 107
  factors in bone health maintenance, 108–10
  mineral and vitamin intake for healthy bones, 107–8
  osteoporosis, 104–6
  osteoporosis therapy, 111
Boron
  dosage range, 257
  for osteoporosis prevention, 63, 109
  summary of information on, 63–64
Breast cancer, 115–21
  antioxidants and, 118–19
  birth control pills and, 118, 119
  dietary fat and, 116–17, 162–63, 164
  estrogen and hormone replacement therapies (ERT/HRT) and, 117–18, 124, 126, 128, 129
  mortality, 114
  risks, 119–20
  screening, 121
  tamoxifen for, 179–80, 188
Breast cancer prevention
  CoQ_{10} for, 60
  general advice on, 120–21
  phytoestrogens for, 179–80, 181
  selenium for, 95, 96
  vitamin A (beta-carotene) for, 17, 18, 19, 114, 119
  vitamin C for, 119
  vitamin E for, 49, 119
Breast pain (mastodynia)
  beta-carotene and retinol for, 17, 19
  vitamin E for, 47, 48
Brewer's yeast, chromium in, 72
Buying vitamin/mineral supplements, 9–13
  checklist for, 13
  expiration dates, 11–12
  labels, 10
  natural versus synthetic controversy, 11

Caffeine
  coffee and potassium loss, 94
  effects of, 169–70
  ideas for reducing intake of, 170
  as inositol antagonist, 35
Calcium, 65–69
  dosage range, 257
  for high blood pressure, 67
  for osteoporosis prevention, 66, 84, 107–8, 109
  for premenstrual syndrome, 192–93
  as skin nutrient, 211
  summary of information on, 65–69
Calcium carbonate with vitamin D, 43
Caloric intake, recommended, 260–61
Cancer, 113–21. *See also* Breast cancer; Cancer prevention; Cervical dysplasia
  antioxidants and, 114–15, 118–19
  breast cancer, 115–21
  colon cancer, 30, 65, 67, 113, 114, 179
  copper/zinc ratio and, 75
  defined, 113
  facts, 114
  lung cancer, 17, 19–20, 39, 47, 50, 114, 115
  skin cancer, 20, 113, 114, 199, 200–1, 203
Cancer prevention
  American Cancer Society guidelines on, 155–56
  calcium for, 65, 67

CoQ_{10} for, 60
folic acid for, 30
garlic for, 179
molybdenum for, 89
phytoestrogens for, 179–81
retinoids for, 18–19
selenium for, 95, 96, 114
vitamin A (beta-carotene) for, 17, 18, 19, 114, 119
vitamin C for, 38, 39, 114, 115, 119
vitamin E for, 49–50, 114, 115, 119
Carbohydrates, 159–61, 260
Carpal tunnel syndrome, pyridoxine (B_6) for, 29
Cervical dysplasia
folic acid for, 31
human papillomavirus and, 31, 115
vitamin C for cervical cancer, 31, 39
vitamin E levels and, 51
Checklist for buying vitamin/mineral supplements, 13
Chelation, defined, 10
Cherry spots, 201
Chinese medicine, traditional (TCM)
acupuncture, 225, 231–32
balance philosophy, 226–30
demand for, 225–26
herbology, 232–33
integration of Western medicine with, 230–32
practitioners, 236
as primary health care, 233–35
Chinese women, breast cancer in, 117
Chiropractic, 237–43
acceptance and popularity of, 237–38
chiropractors as first contact physicians, 238–39
choosing a chiropractor, 243
education, 242
facts, 238
first visit to a chiropractor, 241
insurance coverage, 243
patient satisfaction with chiropractic care, 241
problems within scope of, 239–40
Chlamydia pneumonia infection, 175
Chocolate
cravings, 192
as food to limit, 261
Cholesterol
defined, 162
nutritional guidelines on, 260
Cholesterol levels
American Heart Association guidelines on, 158
chromium for lowering, 71–72
garlic and onion for lowering, 178–79
heart disease and, 158, 162, 171
niacin for lowering, 27
vitamin C for lowering, 37, 39
Choline
dosage range, 256
summary of information on, 36
Chromium, 71–73
for athletic performance, 136
for diabetes, 71
dosage range, 257
summary of information on 71–73
for weight loss, 72, 221
Cigarette smokers
beta-carotene for, 17, 19–20
cancer deaths from tobacco use, 113
menopausal symptoms (hot flashes) in, 188
onset of menopause in, 185
osteoporosis and, 109
vitamin C for, 39, 115
vitamin E for, 50, 115
wrinkles and, 199
Cigarettes as things to avoid, 262
Climacteric, defined, 185
Coffee
caffeine as inositol antagonist, 35
effects of caffeine, 169–70
ideas for reducing caffeine intake, 170
potassium loss and, 94

Colds
traditional Chinese medicine for, 234
vitamin C for, 37, 39–40
Collagen
aging and, 198
vitamin C for synthesis of, 37
Collagen injections for wrinkles, 206
Colon cancer
as common cancer in women, 114
mortality, 113, 114
Colon cancer prevention
calcium for, 65, 67
folic acid for, 30
garlic for, 179
Complex carbohydrates, 161, 260
Copper, 75–76
dosage range, 257
as skin nutrient, 212
summary of information on, 75–76
CoQ_{10}, 51, 59–61
Coumadin, warning regarding vitamin K and, 55, 57
Crohn's disease, fish oils for, 147, 149
Cyanocobalamin (B_{12}), 32–33
dosage range, 256
homocysteine levels and, 174–75
summary of information on, 32–33
Cysts, 202

Damiana, 184
DASH (Dietary Approach to Stop Hypertension) diet, 152–53
Dementia, B_{12} deficiency as cause of, 33. *See also* Alzheimer's disease
Depression
as osteoporosis risk factor, 109
St. John's wort for, 184
traditional Chinese medicine for, 235
Dermabrasion for wrinkles, 205–6
Dermis (inner layer of skin), 195, 196–97
DHEA (dehydroepiandrosterone), 189–90
Diabetes
chromium for, 71
as magnesium antagonist, 86
magnesium for, 83, 85
triglycerides and, 162
Diarrhea
potassium depletion and, 94
from vitamin C toxicity, 42
Diet, 151–70
alcohol, 169. *See also* Alcohol
American Cancer Society guidelines, 155–56
American Heart Association eating plan, 155
American Heart Association guidelines on cholesterol levels, 158
amino acids, 158–59
carbohydrates, 159–61
complex carbohydrates, 161
DASH (Dietary Approach to Stop Hypertension) diet, 152–53
exercise and, 135–37
fats, 161–67
protein, 158
recommendations on foods to eat, 261
sodium, 167–68
sugars, 160
U.S. Dept. of Agriculture and U.S. Dept. of Health and Human Services guidelines, 156–57
water, 168–69
Dieting, yo-yo, 218–19. *See also* Weight; Weight loss
Diuretics
as magnesium antagonists, 86
potassium depletion from, 94
Doctors
chiropractors, 237–43
M.D.s who practice traditional Western medicine, 249, 252
osteopathic physicians, 245–47
traditional Chinese medicine practitioners, 236
Dolomite, 68
Dong quai, 182

Dosage table, vitamin and mineral, 255–59

Eccrine glands, defined, 197
Ehlers-Danlos syndrome, vitamin C for, 37
Encyclopedia of Natural Medicine, 180
Ephedrine (diet aid), 221
Epidermis (outside layer of skin), 195–96
Estradiol
 breast cancer risk and, 118, 120
 for premenstrual syndrome, 193
Estrogen. *See also* Estrogen and hormone replacement therapies
 calcium loss and low estrogen levels, 69
 estriol, 189
 as inositol antagonist, 35
 magnesium levels and, 83–84
 osteoporosis risk and, 109
 as osteoporosis therapy, 111
 as pyridoxine (B_6) antagonist, 30
 as vitamin A antagonist, 21
 as vitamin C antagonist, 41
 as vitamin E antagonist, 53
 zinc levels and, 100
Estrogen and hormone replacement therapies (ERT/HRT), 123–29. *See also* Menopause
 advantages and disadvantages of ERT, 125–26
 advantages and disadvantages of HRT, 126
 breast cancer risk and, 117–18, 124, 126, 128, 129
 calcium supplementation and, 107
 for heart disease prevention, 125, 128, 175
 for osteoporosis prevention, 104, 105, 125, 126, 129
 pills, patches, injections, and creams, 127–28
 Premarin estrogen therapy, 124–25, 182
Exercise, 131–45
 aerobic exercise intensity, 137–45
 benefits of, 131–32
 diet and, 135–37
 free radicals and, 9, 50, 136
 heart disease and, 171–72, 175
 heart rate and, 132–33
 Kegel exercises, 133–35
 during menopause, 190
 for osteoporosis prevention, 106, 107, 131
 recommendations, 261
Expiration dates on supplements, 11–12

Fats, 161–67
 cholesterol, 158, 162, 260
 olestra, 117, 165
 monounsaturated fats, 162
 nutritional guideline for, 260
 polyunsaturated fats, 162–63
 saturated fats, 163
 tips for fat reduction, 165–67
 trans-fatty acids, 117, 163–65
 triglycerides, defined, 162
Fat-soluble vitamins. *See also* Vitamin A; Vitamin D; Vitamin E; Vitamin K
 defined, 7
 vitamin A, 17–22
 vitamin D, 43–45
 vitamin E, 47–53
 vitamin K, 55–57
Fennel and anise, 183
Ferritin
 defined, 79
 heart disease and, 80, 258
Fiber, 116, 161, 260
Fibrocystic breast disease
 iodine for, 77
 vitamin E for, 48–49
Fingernails, 207–8
Fish oils, 147–49
Folate. *See* Folic acid
Folic acid, 30–32
 dosage range, 256
 homocysteine levels and, 174–75

summary of information on, 30–32
thiamine absorption and, 25
Food, 151–70
alcohol, 169. *See also* Alcohol
American Cancer Society guidelines, 155–56
American Heart Association eating plan, 155
American Heart Association guidelines on cholesterol levels, 158
amino acids, 158–59
carbohydrates, 159–61
complex carbohydrates, 161
DASH (Dietary Approach to Stop Hypertension) diet, 152–53
exercise and, 135–37
fats, 161–67
protein, 158–59
recommendations on foods to eat, 261
sodium, 167–68
sugars, 160
U.S. Dept. of Agriculture and U.S. Dept. of Health and Human Services guidelines, 156–57
water, 168–69
Woman's Guide nutritional guidelines, 260
Free radicals
defined, 9
exercise and, 50, 136
Fungus, toenail, 208

Garlic and fish oil, 149
Garlic and onion, 178–79
Ginkgo biloba, 184
Ginseng, 182–83
Goiters and seaweed consumption, 77
Goldenseal, 184
Gout, vitamin C and, 42
Gout medications as vitamin B_{12} antagonists, 33
Grape seed extract, 40
Gray hair
aging and, 209
biotin for, 34
as osteoporosis risk factor, 109
PABA for, 34
Green tea, 170
Greenwald, Peter, 116
Gums, vitamin C for healthy, 37

Hair
aging's effect on, 209
anatomy, 208–9
biotin for graying hair, 34
gray hair as osteoporosis risk factor, 109
inositol for healthy hair, 35
PABA for graying hair, 34
Harman, Denham, 9
Health care costs and vitamin supplementation, 2
Heart anatomy, 172
Heart disease, 171–76
as cause of death in women, 171
chlamydia pneumonia infection and, 175
diet and, 155, 173–75
estrogen replacement therapy and, 125, 128, 175
exercise for people with heart risk, 141
heart attack symptoms, 176
iron and increased risk of, 75, 80, 81, 258
mitral valve prolapse, 172–73
Heart disease prevention
B vitamins for, 27, 174–75
beta-carotene for, 18
calcium for, 65, 175
chromium for, 71, 72
CoQ_{10} for, 51, 59–60, 175
exercise for, 131, 175
fish oils for, 147–49
garlic for, 178–79
magnesium for, 83, 85, 175
niacin for, 27
selenium for, 95
vitamin C for, 37, 38–39
vitamin E for, 47, 50–51, 175

Height and Weight Table for women, 219
Herbology, Chinese, 232–33
Herbs, 177–84
  for female disorders, 182–84
  garlic and onion, 178–79
  phytoestrogens, 179–82
High blood pressure
  calcium for, 65, 67
  DASH (Dietary Approach to Stop Hypertension) diet, 152–53
  defined, 173–74
  fish oils for, 148
  garlic for, 178
  ginseng's blood pressure warning, 183
  magnesium for, 83, 85
  potassium for, 93
  sodium and, 167–68
  vitamin D for, 43, 44
Hirsutism, 209–10
Homocysteine, 174–75
Hopkins, Virginia, 194
Hormone replacement therapies (ERT/HRT), 123–29. *See also* Menopause
  advantages and disadvantages of ERT, 125–26
  advantages and disadvantages of HRT, 126
  breast cancer risk and, 117–18, 124, 126, 128, 129
  calcium supplementation and, 107
  for heart disease prevention, 125, 128, 175
  for osteoporosis prevention, 104, 105, 125, 126, 129
  pills, patches, injections, and creams, 127–28
  Premarin estrogen therapy, 124–25, 182
Hospital costs and vitamin supplementation, 2
Hot flashes
  caffeine as trigger for, 169
  estrogen and hormone replacement therapies for, 124, 187
  exercise for, 190
  herbs for, 183
  phytoestrogens for, 190
  in smokers, 188
  vitamin E for, 47, 48, 188
Human papillomavirus
  cervical cancer and, 31, 115
  folic acid as protective agent against, 31
Hypertension. *See* High blood pressure
Hypothyroidism and low levels of riboflavin, 26
Hysterectomy
  hormone therapy after, 124
  testosterone creams after, 128

Imedeen for sun-damaged skin, 204
Incontinence, urinary, 133–35, 210
Inositol
  dosage range, 256
  summary of information on, 35
Iodine
  dosage range, 257
  summary of information on, 77–78
Iron, 79–81
  for anemia, 79
  for athletes, 135, 136
  dosage range, 257
  herbal remedy warnings about iron absorption, 183, 184
  summary of information on, 79–81
  vitamin C for increased absorption of, 42
  as vitamin E antagonist, 53
The Iron Balance, 79
Iron poisoning in children, 81

Jacobowitz, Ruth, 48
Japanese women, breast cancer in, 116, 180

Kandel, Joseph, 237
Kegel exercises, 133–35
Kidney stones
calcium and, 68, 69, 107
vitamin C and, 42
Koch, Robert, 251

Labels, supplement, 10
Lauffer, Dr., 79
Lecithin, choline supplied as, 36
Lee, John R., 194
Licorice root, 183
Lister, Joseph, 250
Liver spots, 202
L-tryptophan, safety issues, 27
Lung cancer prevention
beta-carotene for, 17, 19–20
selenium for, 114
vitamin C for, 39, 115
vitamin E for, 47, 50, 115

Magnesium, 83–86
dosage range, 257
for high blood pressure, 83, 85
for osteoporosis prevention, 84, 109
for premenstrual syndrome, 192–93
summary of information on, 83–86
Manganese, 87–88
dosage range, 258
for osteoporosis prevention, 87, 109
summary of information on, 87–88
Mastodynia
beta-carotene and retinol for, 17, 19
vitamin E for, 47, 48
Medicine, traditional Chinese, 225–36
acupuncture, 225, 231–32
balance philosophy, 226–30
demand for, 225–26
herbology, 232–33
integration of Western medicine with, 230–32
practitioners, 236
as primary health care, 233–35
Medicine, traditional Western
Eastern medicine versus, 226–29
history and description of, 249–52
integration of Chinese medicine with, 230–32
Melanomas, malignant, 114, 199, 201
Memory loss
choline for, 36
ginkgo biloba for, 184
thiamine for, 24
vitamin E for Alzheimer's disease, 47, 51
Menopause, 185–90
defined, 185
early menopause as osteoporosis risk factor, 109
estrogen and hormone replacement therapies, 123–29
hot flashes, 48, 186, 188, 190. *See also* Hot flashes
sexual desire during, 186–87
treatments for menopausal problems, 187–90
Menopause and the Years Ahead, 48
Menstrual pain, herbs for, 182, 183. *See also* Premenstrual syndrome
Minerals. *See also* specific mineral
buying a vitamin/mineral supplement, 9–13
defined, 7
dosage range table, 255–59
Woman's Guide suggestions for a vitamin/mineral supplement, 259–60
women's need for vitamin/mineral supplements, 8–9
Moisturizers, alpha-hydroxy acid, 206–7
Moles (nevi), 202
Molybdenum
dosage range, 258
summary of information on, 89–90
Monounsaturated fats, defined, 162
Murray, Michael, 180

Nails, 207–8
Natural Menopause, 48
Natural versus synthetically derived vitamins, 11
Niacin (B_3)
  dosage range, 256
  summary of information on, 26–28
Niacinamide, 26–27
Nicotinic acid
  defined, 26–27
  for raising high-density lipoproteins (HDLs), 27
  toxicity problems, 28
Night blindness, 17
Nonsteroidal anti-inflammatory drugs as vitamin C antagonists, 41

O'Hanlan, K., 48
Olestra, 117, 165, 175
150 Most-Asked Questions about Menopause, 48
Oral contraceptive users
  beta-carotene levels in, 21
  breast cancer risk in, 118, 119
  cervical dysplasia in, 31
  folate levels in, 32
  vitamin C for, 41
  vitamin E and, 53
Oriental medicine, 236. *See also* Traditional Chinese medicine
Osteoarthritis, vitamin C for, 40
Osteomalacia, vitamin D for prevention of, 43, 44
Osteopathic medicine, 245–47
Osteoporosis
  defined, 104–6
  factors in bone health maintenance, 108–10
  medications that increase risk of, 69
  screening, 110–11
  treatment, 111
Osteoporosis prevention
  boron for, 63, 109
  calcium for, 66, 84, 107–8, 109
  estrogen and hormone replacement therapies for, 104, 105, 125, 126, 129
  exercise for, 106, 107, 131
  fluoride for, 66
  magnesium for, 84, 109
  manganese for, 87, 109
  phosphorus for, 91, 108, 109
  summary of tips for good bone health, 109–10
  vitamin D for, 45, 107, 108, 109
  vitamin K for, 55

Palmer, D. D., 237
PABA. *See* Para-aminobenzoic acid
Pantothenic acid (B_5), 28–29
  dosage range, 256
  summary of information on, 28–29
  for weight loss, 221–22
Para-aminobenzoic acid (PABA)
  dosage range, 256
  summary of information on, 34–35
  sunscreens with, 34, 35, 203
Pasteur, Louis, 250
Pauling, Dr., 41
Pellagra, 7, 27
Pernicious anemia, 33
Perry, S., 48
Phosphorus
  for bone health, 91, 108, 109
  RDA for, 92, 258
  summary of information on, 91–92
Physical activity. *See* Exercise
Physical performance. *See* Athletic performance
Phytoestrogens, 179–82
  beneficial effects of, 180
  defined, 179
  herbs with, 182–83
  for menopausal complaints, 189, 190
Pizzorno, Joseph, 180
PMS. *See* Premenstrual syndrome
Polyunsaturated fats, 162–63
Potassium
  RDA for, 258
  summary of information on, 93–94

Pre-eclampsia, 83, 85
Pregnancy*
calcium and, 66, 69
as Dong quai (phytoestrogen herb) contraindication, 182
as estrogen therapy contraindication, 125
folic acid for prevention of birth defects, 30–31, 32
herbs used during childbirth, 183
magnesium levels during, 84
warning regarding vitamin A and, 22
Premarin estrogen therapy, 124–25, 182
Premenstrual magnification
antidepressants for, 194
defined, 191
Premenstrual syndrome (PMS), 191–94
calcium for, 192–93
defined, 191
magnesium for, 192–93
natural progesterone for, 193, 194
pyridoxine (B_6) for, 29, 192, 193
red raspberries for, 183
therapy, 193–94
traditional Chinese medicine for, 234
vitamin E for, 47, 49, 193
Proanthocyanidins, 40
Progesterone
estrogen replacement therapy and, 125
for menopausal complaints, 128
natural versus synthetic, 126, 193
for premenstrual syndrome, 193, 194
Protein, 158–59, 260
Psoriasis
fish oils for, 147, 149
vitamin A for, 20
vitamin D for, 44
Pyridoxine (B_6), 29–30
dosage range, 256
homocysteine levels and, 174–75
for premenstrual syndrome, 29, 192, 193
summary of information on, 29–30

Raloxifene, 189
Recommended dietary allowances (RDAS), 8, 255–58
Red raspberries, 183
Reed, Walter, 251
Retinoids
for acne, 17, 20, 22
defined, 18
for sun-damaged skin, 20, 204, 205, 212
Retinol
for cancer prevention, 18–19
defined, 18
food sources of, 20
for mastodynia (sore breasts), 19
warning regarding, 21–22
Riboflavin (B_2)
dosage range, 255
summary of information on, 25–26
for women athletes, 136
Rice
polished rice and beriberi, 24
unmilled rice as thiamine source, 25
Rickets, 7, 43
Roper, Susan, 206, 212
Ross, Ronald, 251

Sage, 183
Salk polio vaccine, 251
Sarsparilla, 184
Saturated fats, defined, 163
Scurvy, 7, 42
Seborrheic keratoses, 200
Selective estrogen receptor modulators (SERMS), 111, 188–89
Selenium, 95–97
for cancer prevention, 95, 96
dosage range, 258
summary of information on, 95–97
vitamin E and, 47, 49, 96

*For the U.S. RDA for vitamins and minerals for pregnant and nursing women, see recommendation section for each vitamin or mineral.

Semmelweis, Ignaz, 250
Sexual desire during menopause, 186–87
Shelf-life testing of supplements, 12
Skin, 195–216
  acne, 17, 20, 22
  aging's effect on, 197–98
  anatomy, 195–97
  cancer, 113, 114, 199, 200–1, 203
  hair, 34, 35, 109, 208–10
  laser resurfacing for wrinkles, 206, 212–16
  nails, 207–8
  nutrients and treatments, 211–12
  psoriasis, 20, 44, 147, 149
  smoking's effect on, 199
  spots, keratoses, carcinomas, and moles, 200–2
  sun damage, 198–99
  sun damage prevention and treatment, 202–7
Skin cancer
  basal cell carcinomas, 199, 200
  melanomas, 114, 199, 201
  squamous cell carcinomas, 199, 200–1
  sun exposure and, 113, 199
  sunscreens and, 203
  vitamin A derivatives and, 20
Skin tags, 201
Skin ulcers, vitamin C for, 38, 211
Smokers
  beta-carotene for, 17, 19–20
  cancer deaths from tobacco use, 113
  menopausal symptoms (hot flashes) in, 188
  osteoporosis and, 109
  skin wrinkles and lines in, 199
  vitamin C for, 39, 115
  vitamin E for, 50, 115
Sodium, 167–68
Sodium bicarbonate as riboflavin antagonist, 26
Soybeans, 120, 180–81
Spider veins, 201
Spina bifida, 30–31
Squamous cell carcinomas, 20, 199, 200–1
St. John's wort, 184
Starches, 161
Still, Andrew T., 245
Stress, pantothenic acid (B_5) for, 28
Stroke prevention
  garlic and onion for, 178, 179
  potassium for, 93
  vitamin C for, 38
Subcutis (bottom layer of skin), 195, 197
Sudderth, David, 237
Sulfa drugs
  as biotin antagonists, 34
  as PABA antagonists, 35
Sun damage and aging skin, 198–99
Sun damage prevention and treatment, 202–7
Sunscreens
  PABA, 34, 35, 203
  skin cancer and, 203
  vitamin D synthesis and, 45
Supplements, vitamin/mineral
  advice on buying, 9–13
  Woman's Guide suggestions for, 259–60
  women's need for, 8–9
Sweat glands, 197
Synthetic versus natural vitamins, 11

Tea, 110, 170
Teeth and gums
  calcium for teeth, 65
  enamel damage caused by chewable vitamin C, 42
  osteoporosis and loss of teeth, 105–6
  phosphorus for teeth formation, 91
  sugar and tooth decay, 160
  vitamin C for healthy gums, 37
  vitamin D for for teeth, 43, 44
Thiamine (B_1)
  dosage range, 255
  summary of information on, 24–25

Thyroid function, iodine for, 77
Time-release vitamins, 12
Toenails, 208
Traditional Chinese medicine (TCM)
 acupuncture, 225, 231–32
 balance philosophy, 226–30
 demand for, 225–26
 herbology, 232–33
 integration of Western medicine with, 230–32
 practitioners, 236
 as primary health care, 233–35
Traditional Western medicine
 Eastern medicine versus, 226–29
 history and description of, 249–52
 integration of Chinese medicine with, 230–32
Trans-fatty acids, 117, 163–65, 175
Triglycerides, defined, 162
Tryptophan
 B_6 and riboflavin deficiencies and, 28
 defined, 27
 for premenstrual syndrome, 193
Tuberculosis, vitamin B_6 and drugs for, 30

Ulcerative colitis, folic acid for, 30
Units of measurement for vitamins, 12–13
Urinary incontinence, 133–35, 210

Vaginal and urinary tracts, 210–11
Vaginal dryness, 17, 187, 188, 190
Vaginal estrogen creams, 127
Vaginitis, 160, 210
Vegetarian athletes, 135
Vegetarians
 bone density in, 66
 breast cancer risk in, 120
 cyanocobalamin (B_{12}) deficiencies in, 33
 niacin (B_3) and, 28
 pyridoxine (B_6) and, 30
 zinc levels in, 100
Vitamin A, 17–22
 for breast cancer prevention, 17, 18, 19, 114, 119
 dosage range, 255
 in fish oils, 20, 149
 as skin nutrient, 211
 summary of information on, 17–22
 for vaginal dryness, 17, 188
Vitamin C, 37–42
 for cancer prevention, 37, 38, 39, 114, 115
 for colds, 37, 39–40
 copper and, 75, 76
 dosage range, 256
 summary of information on, 37–42
 for wound healing, 37, 38, 211
Vitamin D, 43–45
 dosage range, 256
 for osteoporosis prevention, 45, 107, 108, 109
 summary of information on, 43–45
Vitamin E, 47–53
 for athletic performance, 135, 136
 for cancer prevention, 49–50, 114, 115
 dosage range, 257
 for heart disease prevention, 47, 50–51, 175
 for premenstrual syndrome, 49, 193
 selenium and, 49, 96
 for skin, 211
 summary of information on, 47–53
 for sunburn, 203–4
 as vitamin A antagonist, 21
Vitamin K, 55–57
 blood thinners and, 55, 57
 dosage range, 257
 summary of information on, 55–57
 vitamin E and, 53, 57
Vitamin/mineral dosage range table, 255–59
Vitamin/mineral supplement, *Woman's Guide* suggestions for, 259–60
Vitamins. *See also* specific vitamins
 antagonists and, 10–11
 bioavailability of, 10

checklist for buying, 13
defined, 7
expiration dates for, 11
natural versus synthetic, 11
need for vitamin supplementation in women, 8–9
when to take, 12
Vivida for sun-damaged skin, 204

Water, 168–69
Water-soluble vitamins. *See also* B vitamins; Vitamin C
B vitamins, 23–36
defined, 7
vitamin C, 37–42
when to take, 12
Weight
ideal body, 217, 218–21
mortality and, 217–18
recommendations on, 261
Weight loss
chromium picolinate for, 72, 221
pantothenic acid for, 221–22
sugar reduction for, 160
wrinkles and, 199–200
Wernicke-Korsakoff syndrome, 24
Western medicine
Eastern medicine versus, 226–29
history and description of, 249–52
integration of Chinese medicine with, 230–32
What Your Doctor May Not Tell You About Menopause, 194
Wilson's disease and copper supplementation, 76
Woman's Guide nutritional guidelines, 260–62
Woman's Guide suggestions for a vitamin and mineral supplement, 259–60
Women's health issues
breast cancer, 115–21. *See also* Breast cancer
cancer facts concerning women, 114. *See also* Cancer; Cancer prevention
estrogen and hormone replacement therapies, 123–29
heart disease, 171–76
herbs for female disorders, 182–84
menopause, 185–90
osteoporosis, 104–6. *See also* Osteoporosis
premenstrual syndrome, 191–94
vitamin and mineral supplementation, 8–9
weight, 217–22
Wrinkles
alpha-hydroxy acid moisturizers for, 206–7
collagen injections for, 206
dermabrasion for, 205–6
estrogen and hormone replacement therapies and, 127
laser resurfacing for, 206, 212–16
Retin-A and Renova for, 204, 212
smoking and, 199
weight loss and, 199–200

Yams, 181, 189
Yellow Emperor's Inner Classic, 232
Yogurt
for breast cancer prevention, 121
low-fat, 166
vitamin K synthesis and, 56

Zinc, 99–100
for athletes, 135, 136
cancer and, 75
copper status and, 75, 76, 100, 259
dosage range, 258
as skin treatment, 212
summary of information on, 99–100
Zinc picolinate, 10, 258

About the Authors

SHERRY WILSON SULTENFUSS, M.S., is a writer and researcher interested in women's health.

Thomas J. Sultenfuss, M.D., is a board-certified dermatologist. Together they completed *A Woman's Guide to Vitamins and Minerals* in 1995.

This second edition, *A Woman's Guide to Vitamins, Minerals, and Alternative Healing*, updates and expands on the original information with the most recent research. It also includes information about acupuncture, chiropractic, osteopathic, and allopathic medicine. This book can help women choose the right foods to eat, know the right vitamins, minerals, and herbs to take, and learn the real facts about acupuncturists and chiropractors.